But I'm Hungry!

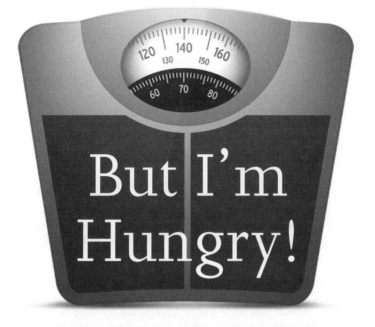

But I'm Hungry!

2 STEPS TO BEATING HUNGER AND LOSING WEIGHT FOREVER

By Marie Suszynski
and
Crystal Petrello, MS, RD

Edited by Sue Mellen

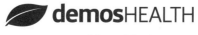

New York

Visit our website at www.demoshealth.com

ISBN: 978-1-936303-49-6
e-book ISBN: 978-1-617051-69-2

Acquisitions Editor: Noreen Henson
Compositor: diacriTech

The scale image is courtesy of Windows Clip Art.

Medical information provided by Demos Health, in the absence of a visit with a health care professional, must be considered as an educational service only. This book is not designed to replace a physician's independent judgment about the appropriateness or risks of a procedure or therapy for a given patient. Our purpose is to provide you with information that will help you make your own health care decisions.

The information and opinions provided here are believed to be accurate and sound, based on the best judgment available to the authors, editors, and publisher, but readers who fail to consult appropriate health authorities assume the risk of injuries. The publisher is not responsible for errors or omissions. The editors and publisher welcome any reader to report to the publisher any discrepancies or inaccuracies noticed.

Library of Congress Cataloging-in-Publication Data

Suszynski, Marie Elaina.
   But I'm hungry!: 2 steps to beating hunger and losing weight forever/by Marie Suszynski and Crystal Petrello, MS, RD; edited by Sue Mellen.
      pages cm
   Includes index.
   ISBN 978-1-936303-49-6 (pbk.)—ISBN 978-1-61705-169-2 (e-book) (print)
      1. Weight loss—Popular works. 2. Reducing diets. 3. Eating well. I. Petrello, Crystal.
II. Mellen, Sue. III. Title.
   RM222.2.S889 2013
   613.2'5—dc23
                           2012029938

Special discounts on bulk quantities of Demos Health books are available to corporations, professional associations, pharmaceutical companies, health care organizations, and other qualifying groups. For details, please contact:

Special Sales Department
Demos Medical Publishing, LLC
11 West 42nd Street, 15th Floor
New York, NY 10036
Phone: 800-532-8663 or 212-683-0072
Fax: 212-941-7842
E-mail: rsantana@demosmedpub.com

Printed in the United States of America by Bang Printing.

12 13 14 15 / 5 4 3 2 1

Contents

*When you understand how hunger works, you have a better
chance of controlling it.*

*Discover how emotional eating can scuttle your
weight-loss plans.*

*Learn how to read and react to the satisfaction signals your
body telegraphs.*

*Learn how exercise can help you burn off the 3,500 calories
stored in every pound of fat and keep hunger in check by
suppressing your appetite.*

Learn how to get ready for successful weight loss.

About the Authors

Marie Suszynski is a long-time health writer in Pennsylvania. She writes for online publications such as Everyday Health and WebMD and has been a contributing writer for more than a dozen books by *Prevention* magazine and other publishers. She also covered the insurance industry as a reporter for an online newswire and print newsletter published by the A.M. Best Co.

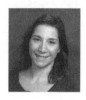

Marie is originally from the Buffalo, NY, area. She received her bachelor's degree from the University at Buffalo, State University of New York, and a master's degree from the Medill School of Journalism at Northwestern University in Evanston, IL.

She has written about everything from diabetes to skin care to mental health, but she has a passion for writing about food, exercise, and weight loss.

Crystal Petrello, MS, RD, is an experienced and accomplished registered dietitian who operates her own dietary consulting company, Crystal Clear Wellness & Nutrition, in Las Vegas, Nevada. While serving in the Air National Guard, she earned her bachelor's degree in medical dietetics from The Ohio State University. She later earned her master's degree in community nutrition and health from Ohio University, where she conducted research around how fruit and vegetable consumption reflect perceptions of health and food security.

Throughout the years, her work and volunteer experience has taken her around the world, from Native American reservations in Minnesota to rural hospitals in India. Recently, she served as the Director of Nutrition for a hospital in southern Ohio and later the Managing Dietitian for an Arizona Women, Infants, and Children program.

Crystal has taught classes for the annual Celiac Disease Conference at Nationwide Children's Hospital in Columbus, Ohio. She is a member of the American Dietetic Association, American Diabetes Association, and the American Congenital Heart Disease Association. Crystal is also the Physicians' Committee for Responsible Medicine's Registered Dietician spokesperson for Las Vegas.

Acknowledgments

The *But I'm Hungry!* team would like to thank Noreen Henson at Demos Medical Publishing for believing in this book and working hard to share it with the world. Thank you Dana Bigelow and the other editors at Demos for shaping it into the book it is today.

We are also grateful to the physicians, dietitians, psychologists, and other experts who kindly shared their knowledge and expertise to help us write this book. In addition, we thank the sixteen people who conquered their battles with weight and shared their personal stories, lent guidance, and offered motivation to help our readers triumph and reach their goals.

Our thanks go out to:

- Sheila Abrahams
- Carol Brannan
- Lisa Bunce, RD
- Dan Collins
- Wendy Cornett
- Jennifer Doyle
- Justin Doyle
- Jessica Fishman Levinson, MS, RD
- Jennette Fulda
- Robert A. Gabbay, MD, PhD
- Keri Gans, RD
- Jo Ann Hattner, RD
- Kate Hawley, RD
- Christy D. Hofsess, PhD
- Tracy Jones
- Laura Kendall
- Sally Koller
- Jessica Levinson, MS, RD
- Richard J. Lindquist, MD
- Naomi Lippel
- Bonnie Matthews
- Barbara Mendez
- Heidi Mitchell
- Jackie Newgent, RD
- Robert Oexman
- Melissa Paris
- Theresa Piotrowski, MD
- Robert Proulx
- Judy Simon, RD
- Dana Simpler, MD
- Ellen Stenzel
- Ryan Sullivan
- Bonnie Taub-Dix, RD
- Janice Taylor
- Hoang Uyen X. Nguyen
- Christina Walman
- Amy Wood, PsyD
- H. Theresa Wright, MS, RD, LDN
- Nicolas Wuorenheimo

A big thanks to Shaun Zetlin for all his support and for creating the great exercise quiz for us.

And, finally, we thank our families and friends who supported us from the beginning and throughout the process of creating But I'm Hungry!

Introduction

We're Mad as Hell and We're Not Going to Take It Anymore

Here's why we decided to write But I'm Hungry! We'd heard cries of despair from so many of our friends and clients that the sound—**But I'm Hungry!**—reverberated in our ears. People were tired of being guinea pigs for the massive diet industry as it churned out yet another miracle (read: starvation) diet. They were sick of failing to lose weight and keep it off because fad diets left them feeling hungry and dissatisfied. Duh!!!! If you're hungry all the time you're not going to stick to a diet. (Not unless you have a serious problem with masochism and enjoy going through life accompanied by searing hunger pains.)

So we formed a team—science writer, editor, and registered dietitian—to create a new life/eating plan that would leave people feeling full, satisfied, and energized. Appropriately enough, we named our plan the **Satisfaction Solution**. Not a diet plan, it's a new way of eating and living that can be sustained throughout life. It's all about eating the right foods, in the right portions, and at the right times. Simple.

At root, But I'm Hungry! is about taking back control of your body and health. It's WAY time to wrest that control away from the commercial diet industry (no matter what Jenny Craig says) and make your own healthy, commonsense decisions about what to eat.

And we're here to help with tips, tools and great recipes. Think of us as three BFFs who are always here for you.

Learn

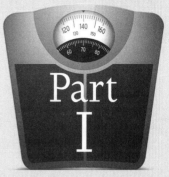

Part
I

That Pesky Hunger

Have you ever thought you could lose weight if you weren't so darned hungry all the time?

Unfortunately, the places we turn to for help don't do the job. How often have you heard that weight loss is as simple as taking in fewer calories than you burn and—voilà!—the pounds will come off?

It's actually a bit more complicated than that. Doctors used to think that a calorie was a calorie. It didn't matter if you ate 1,200 calories in Twinkies all day. If you cut out enough calories, you could lose weight. Now, they're discovering that your body reacts differently to calories that come from different foods.

For one thing, some meals and snacks will make your blood sugar rise and fall like a roller coaster, which triggers your brain to make you feel hungry, even if you've had enough calories. When blood sugar drops very low, nobody has enough willpower to stick to a diet. There's no waiting around to cut up the veggies for a salad. Devouring the ice cream from the freezer is more like it.

Another thing doctors have learned: Some foods literally go straight to your thighs or your tummy, while others are used more efficiently by your body and are less likely to make you fat.

Then there are the tricks the mind plays. We're all born with the natural instincts to know when we're hungry and need to eat and when we're full and need to stop eating. But somewhere along the way our bodies' signals get mixed, maybe because we live in a culture that pushes fatty food twenty-four/seven.

Some people decide to throw in the towel. Life is literally a buffet—with fast-food restaurants on almost every corner and twenty-four-hour grocery stores—and they're going to indulge in everything it has to offer, from Big Macs to triple scoops of ice cream.

But not you. You know overeating doesn't make you happy or healthy. You hold on to the hope that sooner or later you're going to find something that sticks. It's not going to be a fad diet or some crazy scheme to drop twenty pounds in twenty days. It's going to be a plan that fits your life. A way of living and eating that nourishes your body, gives you energy, makes you feel satisfied, and helps you lose weight—finally!

We have the solution. We call it the **Satisfaction Solution**. In these chapters of Part I, you'll learn why you might be feeling so hungry and what you can do to put a stop to hunger once and for all. You'll also find out how to get yourself ready to start losing weight, and that means getting on an exercise schedule, collecting the tools you need, and setting your mind to do this.

After that, in Part II, you'll have a chance to start living it, by following our delicious and satisfying eating plan created by our own dietitian and expert in nutrition, Crystal Petrello, RD. She designed meals and snacks specifically to help you lose weight without feeling deprived. In fact, you'll feel surprisingly satisfied on her eating plan. Then we'll share all of our secrets for losing weight while feeling satiated. These Satisfaction Solution chapters explain how you should be eating and living in order to feel full longer on fewer calories.

Along the way, you're going to read stories of amazing people who have done exactly what you're about to do. In the *What Works for Me* sidebars, you'll hear from others who have lost as little as ten pounds to as many as two hundred pounds. If you feel discouraged and think that you may not be able to do it, get motivation from people who have been in your shoes. And you'll find a ton of nutritional information, healthful tips, and personal musings in Crystal's *Dietitian's Diaries*.

Hunger doesn't have to rule any longer. It's time to beat the beast.

Decoding Hunger

When You Understand How Hunger Works, You Have a Better Chance of Controlling It

What's so hard about losing weight? Cut out 500 to 1,000 calories a day, and in four to seven days you'll be down a pound. Then repeat that ten or twenty or fifty or one hundred times until you've lost the amount of weight you need to lose.

We'll tell you what's so hard about that: hunger.

Our bodies are equipped with powerful processes that drive hunger. If you don't understand them, it's easy to get caught in an endless cycle of eating that keeps you ravenous for more. Not surprisingly, it's very difficult to lose weight under those circumstances [1].

The first step is to understand that it's normal, says Richard J. Lindquist, MD, medical program director, and a bariatric physician at Swedish Weight Loss Services in Seattle, W.A. "You're not broken," Dr. Lindquist tells his patients [1].

And the next step is to learn how your body works to make you feel hungry and then find out how to break the hunger cycle.

Your Appetite: It's More Complex than You Might Think

You would think it would be simple: When your stomach is empty, you're hungry. After you've eaten enough, you won't have the urge to eat anymore. But it's a lot more complicated than that.

There's plenty of misunderstanding about hunger and appetite, even among doctors. "I was taught (and we're often still taught in medical training) that a calorie is a calorie is a calorie," says Dr. Lindquist. "Conventional thinking says that whether it's protein, carbohydrate, or fat, it's treated equally by the body" [1].

5

Following that train of thought, weight control is simply a matter of taking in fewer calories than you burn leads to weight loss. "But that conventional thinking is actually wrong," Dr. Lindquist says [1].

Doctors still don't know all of the factors that are involved in obesity and hunger, but they've pinpointed a few hormones that play a big role [1].

Insulin

Now doctors know that calories from different foods are treated differently in the body. Carbohydrates (carbs), for instance, are converted to glucose, which is a form of sugar that your body uses for energy [1]. After you eat, your blood glucose level (or blood sugar level) goes up, and that triggers your brain to tell your pancreas to start releasing insulin, a hormone that helps usher the glucose into your cells [2].

That process does two things. First, it causes a rise and fall of your blood sugar levels; although a spike in blood sugar turns off your hunger, the urge to eat comes back when your blood sugar falls. Second, it turns on an enzyme that causes your body to store fat and turns off another enzyme that causes fat burning, Dr. Lindquist says [1].

Eat a meal that's full of carbs and not much else—maybe a breakfast of pancakes, sugary syrup, and orange juice—and you might feel hungry again before lunch, despite eating a hefty amount of calories.

This is also how cravings are born. When there's more glucose in your bloodstream, your brain releases serotonin (a chemical that makes you feel good) and dopamine (a chemical that makes you feel pleasure). Getting that natural high from eating certain foods is very powerful reinforcement, Dr. Lindquist says [1]. (Read more about cravings in Chapter 2.)

People who are overweight or obese are more likely to be resistant to insulin, so their bodies will produce more insulin than normal to convert glucose to energy. Because insulin is a fat-storage hormone, having more of it circulating in your blood isn't a good thing [1]. It's this insensitivity to insulin that leads to metabolic syndrome and type 2 diabetes.

A note on insulin and exercise: Exercise can improve insulin resistance by stimulating your muscle to use the glucose for muscle energy rather than storing fat.

Protein and fat, on the other hand, act differently than carbs. Protein is broken down into amino acids, which can be slowly converted to glucose without causing a spike. These amino acids also tell the muscle to make muscle protein rather than to make more fat. Fat is broken down into fatty acids, which are used to make hormones and cell walls, among other things, Dr. Lindquist says. That means eating from those two food groups is key to getting control over the blood sugar cycle, but more about that later [1].

Ghrelin

When your stomach empties, your ghrelin (a hormone that stimulates your appetite) levels rise. But once you eat, ghrelin levels go down, Dr. Lindquist says. Ghrelin is part of the same biological process that causes your stomach to growl and, like blood glucose, it's a very powerful driver of hunger [1].

Researchers have injected ghrelin into both normal-weight and obese people and found that both groups ate more, but the researchers noted that the obese group ate even more than the lean group [3].

When doctors measure ghrelin levels, they have found that people who are obese have low levels of the hormone in their blood. However, losing weight or having weight-loss surgery returns ghrelin levels to normal.

Ghrelin also tends to send fat to your middle, which is the type of fat doctors say can lead to high blood pressure, insulin resistance, and type 2 diabetes [4].

Leptin

This hormone, which was just recently discovered in 1994, is stimulated by your fat cells [1]. Its role is to tell your brain to lower your appetite and increase the amount of energy you burn when you have extra fat stores.

Researchers expected leptin levels to be low in people who are overweight, which might explain why they ate more than they needed, but they found the opposite was true. People who are obese have higher-than-normal levels of leptin in their blood [1].

They also seem to be insensitive to leptin, in much the same way people can be resistant to insulin. Researchers think overeating leads to a disruption in the way leptin works in the body. Rather than it triggering your brain to stop you from overeating, your brain becomes insensitive to leptin levels [5].

Researchers also wonder if leptin could cause levels of ghrelin to drop, but studies have been inconclusive [5].

How to Beat Hunger Hormones

The good news is, you can reset your hunger hormones to help you lose weight and to stop feeling so darned hungry.

Change the Way You Eat Carbs

When your blood sugar is steady and doesn't swing high and low during the day, you'll feel more satisfied between meals and more likely not to overeat. Protein and fat don't break down into glucose; thus, they do not trigger your pancreas to release insulin and start the hunger cycle [1]. That means choosing fruit, legumes, beans, squash, and sweet potatoes over potatoes, bread, rice, and pasta [1].

Also, pairing carbs with protein or fat and choosing high-fiber carbs (e.g., fruit and whole grains) will have a healthier effect on your blood sugar level, allowing it to rise more slowly and preventing it from dropping sharply and leaving you ravenous.

The recipes we provide, along with the eating plans in Part II, all are specifically designed to help control your blood sugar and keep you full between meals.

Fill up on Protein

In addition to helping keep your blood sugar levels steady, protein also is better than carbs at turning off ghrelin, the hormone that stimulates your appetite, Dr. Lindquist says.

A host of research shows that protein makes people feel more satisfied than carbs or fat do. In one study, people who ate a diet that was made up of 30 percent protein reported feeling more satisfied after eating than people who ate a diet with 10 percent protein and more fat. The same happened in a sixteen-week study in which people ate a diet with 34 percent protein compared to those who ate just 18 percent protein [6].

Note: We are in no way advocating a protein-only diet. We are suggesting eating healthy protein as part of a balanced diet to help feel satisfied longer, because protein digests more slowly.

Eating more protein has also been found to help people lose weight and keep it off [6].

> *In addition to helping keep your blood sugar levels steady, protein also is better than carbs at turning off ghrelin, the hormone that stimulates your appetite.*

No worries about how to get more protein. We've done the work for you; following our satisfying eating plan in Part Two will give you the perfect amount of protein to control your hormone levels and help you lose weight without feeling hungry.

Use Hunger as a Guide

You don't have to be starving before you eat, but waiting for the signals from your body to sit down to a meal has been found to lower insulin resistance and lead to less body fat [7].

Researchers told eighty-nine people to eat at the first sign of hunger (but not before) and compared their blood sugar level and insulin sensitivity to those of thirty-one people who weren't trained to listen to their hunger. They found that waiting for the body's cues to eat significantly lowered insulin resistance and prevented blood sugar levels from peaking too high. After five months, those who listened to their hunger signals also weighed less than the other group and had fewer risk factors for cardiovascular disease [7].

The researchers think that eating before your blood sugar has dropped low enough to signal your body to feel hungry leads to a mild case of hyperglycemia when your blood sugar levels are high [7].

Get Your Heart Pumping

Research has shown that getting exercise can lower leptin levels [5] and increase your sensitivity to insulin. Both aerobic exercise, such as walking or cycling, and strength training, such as lifting weights, are important. In a study conducted by researchers at the University of Pennsylvania, overweight or obese women who lifted weights twice a week were better at keeping off belly fat (which leads to insulin resistance) than women who didn't lift at all [8].

Limit High-Fructose Corn Syrup

High fructose, often in the form of high-fructose corn syrup, which you get when you drink regular soda and processed foods, doesn't trigger your body to secrete insulin, and that can lead to interference with your body's leptin and ghrelin levels. When researchers measured the hormone levels of twelve people after eating three meals on two separate days, they found that getting high levels of fructose lowered the amount of insulin and leptin in their blood, but increased ghrelin. That can lead to eating more calories and gaining weight, the study authors reported [9].

High-fructose corn syrup can be found in everything from ketchup to bread, but checking food labels can help you avoid it. Also, reaching more often for fresh fruits, vegetables, and whole grains, rather than relying on processed foods, will help you kick fructose to the curb.

Lose the Weight and the Hunger

Some experts believe that, as soon as you start to lose weight, your hormonal systems will correct themselves, helping you break the hunger hormone cycle, Dr. Lindquist says. Carb cravings decrease once you shift away from a high simple-carbohydrate diet [1].

What Not to Do

Research has found that low-fat, high-carb meals seem to increase leptin levels, which leads to more hunger and weight gain. However, eating more fat at your meals and cutting down on carbs can lower leptin levels.

In the Meantime, Condition Yourself for Weight Loss

As you're resetting your hormones to help you stop feeling hungry between meals, keep in mind what a huge role your mind plays in making you feel hungry, or, rather, making you think you're hungry when you're really not.

"One of the things we understand is that hunger is conditioned," says Dana Simpler, MD, a physician at Mercy Medical Center in Baltimore, Md.

You can condition your body to expect food when it really doesn't need it. "If you always have an after-dinner snack, you've trained your body that it's time again for food and you'll be hungry," she says [10].

Part of the trick to kicking hunger is to stop being afraid of it. When you're afraid of being hungry, you tend to overeat to compensate for something that may or may not happen in the future [8]. You also may eat before you feel hungry, which can lead to higher blood sugar levels, which interferes with your body's natural cues to eat and feel satisfied once you've had enough calories [7].

If you're used to having an after-dinner snack, try taking it out of your schedule. And when you feel the urge to open the fridge, remind yourself that you ate dinner not too long ago, and what you're feeling probably isn't true hunger.

> *Part of the trick to kicking hunger is to stop being afraid of it.*

When you make these small changes, you're probably ready for bigger ones, such as swapping your usual pancake breakfast for one that will better control your hunger.

What Works for Me

Laura Kendall, a cake decorator in Kenmore, N.Y.

I gained weight during my two pregnancies and didn't do much to lose it while raising my two sons, who are now six and three. That doesn't mean I didn't want to lose weight. I did, but I told myself that the way I was eating was just fine. I must have a thyroid problem, I thought, or something else must be going on that's not letting me drop the pounds.

Then I saw my aunt, who had been diagnosed with diabetes, make some lifestyle changes and lose weight. And I watched my brother drop almost one hundred pounds by counting his calories.

At the same time, I started getting scared that I could end up with diabetes. I noticed that carbs were making my blood sugar spike and drop. If I ate a pancake, I'd be shaky in two hours. I couldn't fool myself any longer into thinking my eating habits weren't to blame. It was time to change.

I started with little things. I had never been a big breakfast eater, but I began having an English muffin and an egg or egg white in the morning. In the past, I ate a sandwich for lunch and paired it with chips or another unhealthy snack. Now I have soup with low-fat crackers or a Lean Cuisine meal. Convenience is key because I have my two boys to take care of. If it's prepared and easy to cook in a few minutes, I'm good to go. I also added in plenty of vegetables. Some days lunch might be a plate of sautéed broccoli and mushrooms.

The best part about it was that I barely felt hungry. I focused on getting more food for fewer calories. Rather than slathering margarine on an English muffin, I used spray butter. And because my mornings are the busiest time, I would have lunch at two in the afternoon when I finally had time to focus on food. Because dinner was three hours away, I didn't have time to get hungry before it was time to eat again.

My nighttime eating changed, too. My husband and I had a bad habit of sitting down in front of the television at night with a big bowl of ice cream. I knew that had to stop for me, so I started buying little 100-calorie cups of fat-free, sugar-free lemon ice. I took my time eating it and made it last as long as it took him to finish off his giant bowl of ice cream. Sweet and satisfying, it was the perfect fix.

In the first two weeks of making these changes, I lost ten pounds. That was motivation to keep it up. After that I consistently lost about two pounds a week for the next six months, and then my weight loss slowed to one pound a week.

Nine months after I set my mind to lose weight, I was fifty-seven pounds lighter.

And to be honest, I cheated along the way. People ask me how I did it and my answer is: I cheat. Burgers and fries are my favorite things in the world, so I have them once in a while. However, I notice that I get full faster now that I'm used to eating lighter meals. I no longer polish off the entire plate. Instead, I really listen to my body and stop eating when I'm satisfied. The next day, I go right back to my new, healthy eating habits.

How Long Does Food Stay in Your Stomach?

Considering that nutritionists recommend eating every two to four hours to stave off hunger, you would think food empties from the stomach that quickly. But it actually takes six to eight hours for food to make its way through your stomach and small intestine after you eat. Then it heads into your large intestine or colon. It can take up to twenty-four hours, or even days, before undigested food gets eliminated from your body [11].

Why It's Worth the Fight

If you have some pounds to lose, you probably already have your reasons for wanting to slim down, whether it's fear of developing diabetes, wanting to fit into an airplane seat, or simply feeling better.

But if you need more convincing, here are some benefits you may not have thought of.

- You'll reset your hormone levels so hunger will be less of an issue [1, 12].
- Your joints will feel better. Every pound of weight you lose takes four pounds of pressure off your knees [13].
- If you have diabetes, losing just ten to fifteen pounds can help you lower your blood sugar levels [14].
- If you have high blood pressure or high cholesterol, you can watch your levels drop significantly [15].
- You'll lower your risk of heart disease, stroke, and some cancers [16].
- You'll calm the burn of acid reflux [16].
- You'll have more energy than you've had in years.
- You'll think more clearly, according to a study that found people of normal weight scored better on cognitive tests than people who were overweight [17].
- If you play sports like tennis or basketball, you'll probably see an improvement in your game [17].
- You'll be able to walk, run, bike, hike, or ski longer.
- You'll take risks. Losing weight will give you confidence, and that may mean you'll try something daring, like skydiving or going after your dream job [17].
- You'll meet new friends at the gym or in support groups.
- You'll sleep better. People who have sleep apnea breathe better at night after they lose weight [17].

- Chairs will feel bigger and airplane seats won't feel so tight.
- *Skinny jeans* won't be a banned phrase.
- You'll climb stairs without getting winded.
- Your family may pick up some of your new healthy habits—and get healthier themselves.
- You'll feel more in control of your health and your life.
- Romps in the bedroom may become steamier. Studies have found that people who lose weight report having better sex [18].

You'll get more satisfaction from your food because you'll eat in a more mindful way, savoring every bite [17].

Dietitian's Diary

Welcome!

Once you decide to follow the But I'm Hungry! plan, you are going to learn about yourself in many new and positive ways. By overcoming challenges and succeeding, you'll see just how strong you really are, and you'll feel good about yourself after every meal and at the end of every day.

We'll give you the tips, facts, tools, and motivation you need to beat hunger forever. That doesn't mean you won't slip every now and then along the way, or that you'll never feel hungry again. But hunger will cease to hold you in its grip, so you'll never have to be afraid of it again.

This is a journey, and don't be afraid that you might fail along the way. From here on out, use failure as a growth tool. Remember, it took awhile to gain the weight. It is going to take some life changes and time to lose it. But soon you'll be able to enjoy the fruits of your labor of love.

Recipes

BEAN CHILI MAC   Serves: 8

1 tablespoon canola oil
1 yellow onion, diced
2 teaspoons chili powder
1 teaspoon cumin
1 teaspoon oregano, dried
2 cups water
1 15 oz. can pinto beans, drained and rinsed
1 15 oz. can tomatoes, canned, do not drain
1 tablespoon liquid smoke
1 cup tomato sauce
1 cup TVP (textured vegetable protein)
2 ½ cups whole-wheat pasta, cooked

Directions:

1. Boil water and cook whole-wheat pasta while preparing remaining ingredients.

2. In a large soup pan, sauté onion in heated canola oil until translucent.

3. Add remaining ingredients to the pan and bring to a simmer.

4. Simmer for 20 minutes.

5. Drain pasta well and stir into chili mixture.

6. Serve while hot and add extra chopped raw onions for added kick.

Per serving: 202 calories, 2.5 g fat, 33 g carbohydrate, 4 g fiber, 12 g protein.

BRIE AND PEAR SANDWICH   Serves: 2

½ medium Bosc pear, sliced
2 ounces brie
2 ounces turkey breast, oven roasted, deli thin
2 large sandwich thins
⅛ cup cranberries, dried
⅛ cup apple cider vinegar
juice from medium lime

Directions:

1. On the stovetop, in a small saucepan, heat vinegar and lemon juice.

2. Add cranberries and heat through until berries are plump and most of liquid is gone.

3. Build each sandwich from the bottom up:
    A. Half a sandwich thin
    B. Half of cranberry sauce
    C. 1 ounce brie
    D. Turkey
    E. Pear slices
    F. Other half of sandwich thin

TIP
Place the cheese on top of the warm cranberry sauce to help melt cheese.

Per serving: 327 calories, 10.9 g fat, 35 g carbohydrate, 7.2 g fiber, 21.9 g protein.

NOTE: To make vegetarian, omit meat and add another ounce of cheese.

LIME SHRIMP TACOS   Serves: 4

8 jumbo shrimp, deveined and shell removed
4 tablespoons Mrs. Dash Fiesta Lime Blend
1 cup red onion, diced
4 Roma tomatoes, chopped
1 cup cilantro, chopped
1 yellow bell pepper, diced
1 orange bell pepper, diced
1 cup jicama, diced
8 corn tortillas
Sea salt, to taste

Directions:

1. Butterfly shrimp and sprinkle both sides evenly with Mrs. Dash.

2. Heat tortilla according to package.

3. Mix together onion through jicama in a bowl.

4. In each tortilla place one jumbo shrimp and vegetable mix.

Per serving: 281 calories, 3.6 g fat, 38.6 g carbohydrate, 3.1 g fiber, 23.6 g protein.

What Your Body Needs vs. What You Think It Needs

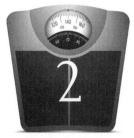

Discover How Emotional Eating Can Scuttle Your Weight-Loss Plans

We tend to eat for hunger only about 15 percent of the time, experts say [1]. The rest of the time, we eat because we're happy or sad or angry or anxious. Or because we're at a restaurant or a party. Or because it's the time of day that we usually eat, or there's still food on our plate. Or because we saw a commercial for a new pizza, or we pass a Dunkin' Donuts on the way to work every day. The bottom line is, we are eating emotionally and not to satisfy our need for nourishment.

Hunger pushes us to fuel our bodies with food. Satiety happens when our fuel gauge is just full enough—not overfull, says Christy D. Hofsess, PhD, licensed psychologist and assistant professor in the Department of Counseling and Health Psychology at Bastyr University in Kenmore, W.A. [2].

It sounds like a perfect internal system to keep our bodies lean and healthy. The problem is, there are at least one hundred and one things that can confuse hunger signals, and it's all too easy to ignore satiety cues.

> "We overeat because of packages, plates, brand names, shapes, smells, and distractions."
>
> Dr. Hofsess [2].

Not to mention our own unique histories with food.

But you don't have to let your environment or your emotions keep you eating past the point of feeling full. Find out how to give your body exactly what it needs to be satisfied, without going overboard.

Crazy Concept: Food as Nourishment

With so much white noise surrounding food and your perception of what you need to eat to feel satisfied, it's easy to forget the right way to fuel your body.

Your body needs carbohydrates, protein, healthy fats, fruits, and vegetables. Getting the nutrients those foods provide is the essence of feeling satisfied.

Your body needs vitamins and minerals from apples, melons, oranges, pears, blueberries, cherries, avocados, greens, broccoli, spinach, cabbage, tomatoes, squash, potatoes, carrots, nuts, beans, legumes, yogurt, whole-grain bread, brown rice, salmon, shrimp, codfish, tofu, olive oil, canola oil, and all of the rest of healthy, natural, whole foods that are available to you [3].

People who eat to nourish their bodies feel more satisfied after eating and aren't as likely to reach for a candy bar when stress strikes.

Notice that your body doesn't *really* need jelly beans, salty chips, or fried foods, and yet they're a staple of many people's lives. We don't advocate abstaining from eating those foods because they may help you feel psychologically satisfied. But your focus should be on the healthy foods that are going to give you ultra-filling nourishment.

Then there's the matter of how much food you need. It varies based on your own metabolism, but there are a couple of websites where you can plug in your age, sex, height, weight, and activity level to find out how many calories you need a day to maintain your weight (go here: http://www.bcm.edu/cnrc/caloriesneed.htm, or here: http://www.mypyramid.gov/mypyramid/index.aspx.) [4, 5].

To lose weight, you'll have to eat 250 to 500 calories less a day to lose up to a pound a week [4].

Keep in mind that there are certain times in life when people need more calories, including children and adolescents who are growing, women who are pregnant or breastfeeding, and people who are suffering from diseases that leave their immune systems compromised. Sometimes caloric intake needs go up before or after surgery, as well [6].

If you're a healthy adult who's ready to change the way you eat to lose weight, there's no need to do a lot of math and planning to figure out how to get the right number of calories and nutrients. In Part II of this book we'll lay out eating plans that will help you start losing weight.

Losing the Urge to Eat When You're Not Hungry

Even when you know what and how much you should be eating, breaking old habits isn't easy, especially when your environment sends you messages to overeat or to choose processed foods that don't nourish your body. Emotional eating—when feelings of anger, sadness, anxiety, loneliness, boredom, or joy send us on a binge—is also a major issue for many people.

And the worst thing about it: You may be so used to reaching for food under certain circumstances that you don't even realize you're doing it.

You can't change your behavior unless you see it for yourself, so the first thing you need to do is recognize when you're not using your internal cues of hunger to eat, says Theresa Piotrowski, MD, medical director of the Medical and Surgical Weight Loss Center at the Lahey Clinic in Boston [1].

It can take up to three months just to recognize that a fight with your husband always sends you to the freezer for a big bowl of ice cream. Then, it can take up to a year to change the behavior, Dr. Piotrowski says [1].

This is where a food log comes in. Dr. Piotrowski advises writing down:

- What you eat;
- How much you eat of each food;
- How many calories you're consuming;
- How much protein you're eating (to be sure you're getting enough satiating protein to help you lose weight);
- The time of day (to help you schedule your meals);
- Your hunger on a scale of one to ten, with ten being very hungry; and
- Your emotional state at the time you ate.

The notes can be eye opening. "I've had patients say, 'I didn't realize I was drinking as much alcohol as I was,' or that the portions were as large as they were," she says. Often, people are immersed in eating the food before they've even realized how many calories they're consuming [1].

Work on Those Emotions

Recording your emotional state in your food log is important because sometimes it's not hunger or the environment that's driving you to eat—it's your own emotional state. Did you polish off the bag of chips because you were happy, sad, or depressed? If you did, find ways to deal with those emotions without food, Dr. Piotrowski says [1].

We know: Easier said than done. That might mean picking up the phone to call a friend, working off anxiety or anger on the treadmill, or writing in a journal, says Barbara Mendez, RPh, MS, a nutritionist, registered pharmacist, and owner of Barbara Mendez Nutrition.

Here's a good idea: Write down things that you enjoy or that calm you, so you have a go-to list to consult the next time you feel you could eat the wallpaper off the walls [7].

In addition to calling a friend, working out, and writing in a journal, here are some more possibilities for your list:

- Take a bubble bath
- Take a short, brisk walk
- Get a hug from your spouse or child
- Jump rope
- Practice deep breathing
- Give yourself a manicure
- Do a few yoga sun salutations
- Play your favorite playlist on your iPod
- Make a cup of herbal tea or coffee
- Scream into a pillow
- Let your emotion take a form in your head, then picture letting go of it
- Meditate
- Play with a pet
- Look at family pictures or other snapshots that remind you of a happy time
- Imagine a calming setting, such as the beach or a rose garden
- Read some jokes from a joke book or a joke website you've bookmarked

Sometimes emotional eating can progress into an all-out binge, when you eat and eat and feel like you can't stop. In mere minutes you could eat hundreds of calories. Once you're in binge mode, it's almost impossible to stop eating, Mendez says [7]. Researchers suspect people who binge have unbalanced brain chemicals that drive hunger, appetite, and digestion and may lead to binges [8].

Bingeing can be a vicious cycle. It leads to guilt, which can lead to feelings of depression, which can lead to more emotional eating and even more binging. People who binge regularly are at higher risk for health problems like high blood pressure and cholesterol, type 2 diabetes, heart disease, gallbladder disease, and some kinds of cancer. People who binge are also more likely to experience anxiety and depression [9].

If you're one of those people who know how you should be eating and you're not doing it, it might be worthwhile to see a therapist who specializes in eating disorders. Make the appointment if you spend a lot of time thinking about food and your weight, and especially if food interferes with your work or your relationships, suggests Amy Wood, PsyD, a psychologist in private practice in Portland, Maine, and author of *Life Your Way*. But, because eating is such a huge part of our culture, most therapists will be able to help you with it, she says [10].

The advantage is that you'll go right to the heart of your issues and finally get freedom from using food to feed emotions, Mendez says [7].

What Works for Me

Wendy Cornett, a freelance writer and editor in Canal Winchester, OH

I've always been conscious about the foods I eat and have led a healthy life. But when my kids were three and nine, I found myself a little heavier than I wanted to be.

My husband and I went on a fantastic cruise with a group of friends and neighbors, and I looked around at the other women wearing their two-piece bathing suits, while I wore a one-piece. I knew I could get my body in bikini shape—the challenge was to figure out what I was doing that wasn't working.

I was eating a vegetarian diet, as I had for twenty years. And I started doing a fifty-five-minute Jillian Michaels workout about three times a week. My weight wasn't budging and I felt exhausted. My knees were so sore as I walked up and down the stairs of my split-level house that I had to ice them regularly.

Something had to change, and I had an idea. I would give my knees a rest and do a thirty-minute workout five days a week first thing in the morning before my kids woke up. Even if I put in a longer DVD, I stopped it after thirty minutes. I loved the consistency of having me-time every morning, and the shorter workouts were much easier on my knees, so I was better able to keep up the routine.

At the same time, I've always been good about getting healthy protein in my diet, and I continued to eat well. As a vegetarian, I knew I had to be conscious of not carbing out (eating too may carbs). Eating a banana, yogurt, berries, and granola in the mornings keeps me satisfied through lunchtime.

By being more consistent with my workout, I lost a good ten pounds, from August to December, bringing my weight down to about 130. I just turned forty-four, and I feel great. My knees don't bother me anymore, and I have more energy. It's been a complete turnaround.

Using Your Noggin: Become a Mindful Eater

Keeping a food log and paying attention to your emotions are two ways to be more mindful about the way you're eating. Another way is to look at the ways you've been conditioned to eat.

When you indulge in a bucket of buttery popcorn every time you go to the movies, you'll probably start feeling hungry for it while you're standing in line to buy your movie ticket, or even when you first have the idea to see a movie.

The same thing can happen at home. Did you polish off a bag of chips simply because you were sitting in front of the television and you have a habit of snacking while watching TV?

Those habits will take real effort to change, but it can be done.

Change the Cues

If you eat in front of the television, rearrange the furniture in the room and sit in a different chair so you can stop associating eating with when you watch TV, Dr. Piotrowski says [1]. Another option: Keep hand weights next to the TV, and do some exercises while you watch. Eventually, you'll lose the urge to eat and gain the urge to exercise when you're in front of the television.

The same goes for other situations. If it's hard to resist the lure of the donut shop you pass on your way to work, take a new route. To kick the movie popcorn habit, go to a different theater, or hit the drive-in instead.

Fill Up on Nutrient-Rich Foods

When you're eating high-quality foods, you'll feel satisfied and are less likely to feel the need to eat when you come face to face with a foot-long hot dog at the ballpark [2].

And once you get a taste for a big, crisp salad full of veggies and grilled salmon, a platter of salty nachos and cheese may not be as appealing as it once was, particularly because you know it won't make you feel as good as you would after eating a healthy meal [10].

Understand the Game

We live in a culture that promotes emotional eating, Dr. Wood says. Food is advertised in an emotional way, telling us we deserve to give ourselves a treat, she says [10].

> Eventually, you'll lose the urge to eat and gain the urge to exercise when you're in front of the television.

It's hugely profitable for companies to sell food, especially food that's cheap to make, so they're going to do everything they can to get you into their restaurants, whether it's by putting a picture of a cupcake in an online ad to stare at you while you read news articles, erecting a highway billboard with bigger-than-life burgers, broadcasting the radio jingle for a fast food restaurant that your child sings for the rest of the day, or creating an avalanche of television and print ads [10].

Even people who don't have food issues fall for it, Dr. Wood says. But if you're particularly sensitive to the lure of greasy onion rings, it's even easier to give in when advertisers are throwing them at you at every turn. The solution can be as simple as being mindful of those messages. Before you get into your car and head to a burger joint, ask yourself if you really want to eat that burger [10].

That doesn't mean you should over-think every piece of food that goes into your mouth, but trust your own intuition about the foods you should be eating rather than letting an advertisement tell you that you need it, Dr. Wood says [10].

Give Yourself Permission

Your answer to whether or not you want to eat the burger may very well be yes, and that's okay. Normal eating sometimes means letting yourself splurge on a burger or eating buffalo wings while watching the Super Bowl, Dr. Hofsess says. The difference is that you're *aware* of eating the food, rather than eating it mindlessly. And when you're aware, you can pay attention to feelings of satiety and perhaps eat two-thirds of what you would normally eat, she says [2].

Savor Every Bite

People who have dieted their entire lives are doing themselves a disservice, Dr. Wood says. Diets tend to label food as good or bad, and when you do that you take away the enjoyment of sinking your teeth into something that gives you pleasure. How about this: instead of telling yourself you can't have your favorite lasagna, sit down to a plate of it, smell it, eat it slowly, taste it, and savor it. When you feel satisfied, push your plate away, knowing you had exactly what you wanted and that you allowed yourself to enjoy it [10].

Keep at It

It takes a lot of practice to eat mindfully. Relapses are a normal part of life. For most people, it takes about forty days to develop a new habit, but there are so many things that can interfere that it's normal to find yourself slipping up [10].

"Give yourself time," Dr. Wood says. "Understand that there are moments, days, and weeks when things are going to be stressful." When you get off track, work on getting back on. Don't beat yourself up about it. Just keep trying [10].

Cravings!

Forget emotions and environmental cues. Sometimes you get a distinct craving for something particular totally out of the blue. And when cravings strike, it's almost always for high-calorie, high-fat foods like potato chips, French fries, and chocolate [11].

Researchers have found that cravings are steeped in imagery. Craving an ice cream sundae? Odds are you can vividly picture the scoops of ice cream nestled in the dish, the hot chocolate sliding down the sides, the airy whipped cream, and the bright red cherry sitting on top [12].

Studies have also found that once you have an image in your head, it's hard to get it out. And it takes mental energy, which means you have a hard time thinking about anything else. People take longer to finish math problems when they're craving chocolate [12].

What do you do about it?

Ride the Wave

Sometimes all it takes to get past a craving is acknowledging that you're having a craving and telling yourself you're not going to give in [2].

If you have an all-or-nothing attitude about cravings, then it's easy to think that if you don't give in, the craving will build up until you explode. "It turns out that it doesn't happen that way," says Dr. Lindquist [13].

Find a Good Distraction

Although imagining a food you're craving can make it hard to focus on work, studies have found that you can think about other things to lose the food cravings. For instance, when study participants imagined a rainbow or the smell of eucalyptus, their food cravings felt less intense [12].

A brisk walk may be your ticket to forgetting about your craving. In a study that involved twenty-five people who usually ate chocolate every day, researchers had them abstain from eating their favorite sweet snack for three days. And walking briskly for just fifteen minutes helped them forget about the chocolate [14].

Here's one healthy, guilt-free way to satisfy a chocolate craving: buy a high-quality dark chocolate.

Get the Taste from a Healthier Food

Sometimes you can satisfy a craving by substituting something healthier for what you're actually craving. Fruity herbal teas might satisfy a sweet tooth. Or a 100-calorie bag of chocolate-covered pretzels or cup of chocolate pudding may keep you from eating an 800-calorie brownie sundae at an ice cream shop [6].

Here's one healthy, guilt-free way to satisfy a chocolate craving: Buy a high-quality dark chocolate. A recent study found that when people who had high blood pressure ate thirty calories worth of dark chocolate every day, their blood pressure improved [15].

Give in Some of the Time

If you tell yourself you can't eat something, you set yourself up for a deprivation binge, Dr. Piotrowski says. Some people have done this their entire lives, she says. It's healthier to allow yourself to have it but to watch your portion. Have a scoop of ice cream instead of a big bowl [1].

Another way to do this: allow yourself to have a cheat day or a cheat meal, Dr. Lindquist says. It's not what you do once in a while that causes problems; it's what you do most days that brings long-term success [13].

Lose the Guilt

Everyone has cravings. Instead of feeling guilty about them, it's better to accept that they're a part of life, and they're probably not going to go away. People who are successful at weight loss give in to cravings occasionally. An urge to dive into a bag of potato chips isn't the end of the world [11].

An Easy Fix: Spare Some Calories from Your Cup

Before you pour yourself another tall glass of sweetened tea, consider this: research has found that the more calories Americans drink, the higher the obesity rate climbs. Even more importantly, that sweet drink isn't going to leave you satisfied [16].

We consume 150 to 300 more calories a day than we did thirty years ago, and half of that is in the form of beverages [16]. Add a daily raspberry iced tea to your diet at 216 calories a bottle, and you'll gain a pound from liquid calories alone in just sixteen days [17].

In a 2009 study from the *American Journal of Clinical Nutrition*, researchers set out to measure the effect liquid calories had on 810 people's weight over eighteen months. Each participant cut 100 calories from his or her diet. Those who took liquid calories out—sugary drinks in particular—lost significantly more weight than those who cut calories from solid food [16].

Taking out liquid calories such as milk, coffee, tea, alcohol, and other drinks led to weight loss, but only lowering the amount of sugary drinks like soda resulted in significant weight loss [16].

Why? Researchers suspect it's because liquid calories aren't satisfying, and you already know how sugar makes your blood sugar levels rise and drop steeply, making you feel hungry soon after. Also, getting a large amount of sugar over time helps promote fat storage [16].

Why Diet Soda Isn't the Answer

It seems like it's a no-brainer. In the mood for a sweet drink, grab a diet soda or diet juice. You'll get the satisfaction of drinking something that tastes like sugar, but without a single calorie.

If only it were that simple. A 2008 study on rats found that diet drinks interfere with the body's ability to predict how many calories it has ingested. Animals (and humans) judge sweet-tasting foods and drinks to have more calories, but drinking zero-calorie beverages that still taste sweet takes away the body's ability over time to gauge how many calories it has consumed [18].

When researchers gave rats sugar or saccharin, they found that the rats that were given the artificial sweetener ate more calories and gained weight [18].

Dietitian's Diary

Emotional Eating

Let's say you are at work and you grab a donut from the conference room. You begin eating the tasty treat, even though you did not feel a sensation of hunger before you picked it up. At some point during the devouring, you ask yourself: "Why am I eating this?" This dialogue is where weight loss starts. Why are you craving a sweet tasty snack an hour after breakfast? Is it that you just found out the project you thought was due tomorrow is actually due today at noon? Are you feeling sad because your family pet just passed on? Or are you just feeling defeated because you have already given up on your morning workouts?

Don't feel alone. It is estimated that 75 percent of overeating is caused by emotions! [19] We ignore our hunger cues and try to bury the loneliness, sadness, and negative feelings with food. To make ourselves feel better about life situations, we tell ourselves we NEED comfort food. Comfort food reminds us of happy memories or simply puts us in a state of ecstasy with the flavor and texture as we chew. I indulge in chocolate or macaroni and cheese myself. On the other hand, there are times we eat because we are happy. We eat to celebrate finishing that project, winning at the casino (especially when they give you a complimentary trip to the buffet), or as we usher in another year of our lives.

I am by no means implying that enjoying food is bad. It is human nature to enjoy food. It is when we use food as our main emotional outlet that we start to see the pounds pile on. I have seen people gain twenty pounds or more from a variety of situations that led to emotional eating.

The first step to controlling emotional eating is recognizing that you are not hungry. Then fess up, not necessarily to others, but definitely to yourself (see Chapter 7 for more on journaling), and acknowledge what is causing these emotions. Once you know the cause, you can begin dealing with your emotions, stress, or whatever it is driving you to seek solace with food in a way that is positive. Cope with and work through your emotions in a way that does not involve food. You can try going for a walk, reading a book, journaling, or maybe by starting to plan a vacation.

Just don't cry over your chocolate cake!

Sugar Substitutes

For some people, sugar substitutes are synonymous with weight loss and enjoying sweet treats without the calories that sugar provides. In terms of nutrition, we are going to focus on their effect on our overall nutrition and hunger satisfaction.

There are two main categories of these fake sugars: artificial sweeteners and sugar alcohols. The difference between artificial sweeteners and sugar alcohols is that artificial sweeteners do not contain calories and sugar alcohols do. In terms of regular sugar, the sugar alcohols have half the amount of calories as the old standby.

It is worth noting that many of these artificial sweeteners are created by a combination of naturally occurring chemicals [20]. It is the process in which they are generally developed, a multi step science-lab process, that makes them subject to scrutiny. All of the following sweeteners are generally recognized as safe or approved as food additives by the Food and Drug Administration (FDA) [20]. Based on recent research, it is the stance of the American Dietetic Association, the authority on all things nutrition, that "consumers can safely enjoy a range of nutritive and non-nutritive sweeteners when consumed in a diet that is guided by current federal nutrition recommendations, such as the Dietary Guidelines for Americans and the Dietary Reference Intakes, as well as individual health goals" [20, p. 255]. Whether or not the sweeteners contain calories, we should consider using them in moderation while following a healthy diet. It is more important to make sure we are eating all the nutritious foods before we eat our sweets. Remember when your mother said you couldn't have dessert until you ate your vegetables? As usual, she was right!

Artificial Sweeteners

Artificial sweeteners are considered non-nutritive because they do not have calories, and they create a sweet flavor without adding much volume to food [20].

Brand Name(s)	Also Known As	How Much Sweeter Than Sugar?
Truvia	Stevia	**200 times
Splenda	Sucralose	**600 times
Sweet'N Low, Sweet Twin, Necta Sweet	Saccharin	**200–700 times
Equal, Nutrasweet, Sugar Twin	Aspartame	**160–220 times
Sunnett, Sweet One, Sweet & Safe	Acesulfame-K	**200 times

Sugar Alcohols

A label can read "sugar-free" when there are sugar alcohols in the food. This is because it replaces sugar, but it is not sugar. It is important to remember that sugar-free does not mean calorie free. In general, sugar alcohols provide half the amount of calories (2 kcal/gram) than sugar (4 kcal/gram) [20]. Contrary to artificial sweeteners, since sugar alcohols contain calories, they are called nutritive sweeteners. They have more of a function than just adding taste to our food. In food production, they help make food look more appetizing [21].

Sugar alcohols are not entirely absorbed, and the parts that are, are absorbed slowly. This causes fermentation in the intestine [22]. If too much is consumed, stomach issues such as gas and diarrhea can result [20].

Types

Name	Kcal/gram	How Much Sweeter Than Sugar?
D-Tagatose	1.5	75–92%
Erythritol	0.2	60–80%
Isomalt	2	45–65%
Lactitol	2	30–40%

Name	Kcal/gram	How Much Sweeter Than Sugar?
Maltitol	2.1	90%
Mannitol	1.6	50–70%
Sorbitol	2.6	50–70%
Trehalose	4	45%
Xylitol	2.4	Same sweetness as sucrose

Hunger Satisfaction

Many people like non-nutritive sweeteners because they make those guilty foods we crave feel a little less guilty, and can make foods we don't love, taste a little better [23]. Studies have shown that non-nutritive sweeteners do not increase appetite and food intake [24]. However, even with the availability of these lower calorie products, as a nation, we keep getting fatter. What gives? Has our perception of sweetness changed with the increased use of added sugars (with calories) and artificial sweeteners (with and without calories)? Remember, even if something is labeled "sugar-free" or "diet" does not mean it is calorie free. You are not eating flavored air! In many products, when the fat content is decreased, the amounts of carbohydrates increase, and vice versa. Look at the nutrition label if you don't believe me! The amounts of calories in a sugar-free product tend to be identical to the amounts in the comparable regular product.

The moral: Choose wisely and read the label.

TANGY PEACH AND WHOLE GRAIN SALAD   **Serves: 8**

3 cups brown rice, cooked and chilled
1 15 oz. can corn, drained and rinsed
1 cup almonds, toasted, chopped
1 cup peas, frozen, rinsed with cold water to remove freeze
1 15 oz. can peaches, drained, rinsed, and diced
¼ cup Light Catalina dressing
¼ cup red onion, finely diced
¼ cup fresh cilantro, chopped

Directions:

1. Combine all in serving dish.
2. Serve chilled.

TIP

Try this with different whole grains, such as quinoa or wheat berries. Switch up the dressing, or omit it all together and enjoy the sweetness of the fruit and zing of the onion.

Per serving: 282 calories, 10.9 g fat, 38 g carbohydrate, 2 g fiber, 8 g protein.

SATISFACTION SOLUTION BURRITO   Serves: 4

1 15 oz. can black beans, drained and rinsed
1 medium green bell pepper, chopped
1 cup yellow onion, diced
1 cup tomatoes, canned, drained
1 cup corn kernels, frozen
1 tablespoon cumin
1 medium avocado, mashed
¼ cup cilantro, chopped
4 large whole-wheat tortillas

Directions:

1. Put corn in a colander and run room-temperature water over until frost is gone.

2. Mix all ingredients through corn together.

3. Put ¼ of vegetable mixture in the center of each tortilla.

4. On the side offer ¼ an avocado and some cilantro for each burrito.

Per serving: 423 calories, 9.9 g fat, 67 g carbohydrate, 5.5 g fiber, 16.3 g protein.

SATISFACTION SOLUTION SALAD   Serves: 1

1 cup spinach
1 cup arugula
½ cup canned black beans, drained and rinsed
2 ounces avocados, chopped (¼ cup)
⅛ cup jicama, chopped
⅛ cup orange bell pepper, chopped

¼ cup tomato, chopped
1 tablespoon fresh lime juice

Directions:

1. Combine all ingredients in a bowl.

2. Drizzle lime juice over the salad.

Per Serving: 262 calories, 9.6 g fat, 32.5 g carbohydrate, 4.14 g fiber, 11.45 g protein.

What Satisfaction Feels Like

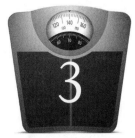

Learn How to Read and React to the Satisfaction
Signals Your Body Telegraphs

Hunger is a physiological drive we can't ignore. Our bodies and brains need fuel to function. If we didn't have this drive to fuel our bodies, we'd grow weak and listless and have trouble thinking straight.

It's not hard to know when you're hungry. But satiety—knowing when you've had enough to eat—is trickier.

Satiety sets in when we've had just enough to eat. Feeling satisfied—or satiated—means gratifying your appetite, says Jackie Newgent, RD, New York City culinary nutritionist and author of *Big Green Cookbook: Hundreds of Planet-Pleasing Recipes & Tips for a Luscious, Low-Carbon Lifestyle* [1].

It's a satisfied feeling that lets us know we've gotten enough calories. But over the years, too many things interfere with satiety, and we lose touch with that feeling of satisfaction. It's due to overeating, consuming too many calories, fad diets, and artificial sweeteners used to try to trick our bodies into losing weight [2].

When we overeat, we're responding to cues outside of our body that tell us to eat, whether the cues are large plates overfilled with food, the people around us who pressure us to have seconds, or eating for comfort [2]. When that happens, we're beyond satisfied by the time we put down our fork. We're stuffed.

Dieting also interferes because it teaches us to ignore the cues our bodies give us, including hunger and satiety. When we're dieting, we eat because the diet says it's time to eat, and we stop eating because the diet tells us that's all we should have. These diets tout self control. But the diets fail because when we start to listen to our body's cues we are hungry on the diet. So, we dive off the wagon and overeat. Then we feel we've failed to control ourselves and overeat again for comfort. The negative cycle begins [2].

According to a survey by the Partnership for Essential Nutrition (a coalition of eleven nonprofit groups that promote healthy diets), nine out of ten Americans surveyed in 2004 were working on maintaining their weight or losing weight. One in five was trying to do that with a low-carb diet. As we will point out in a later chapter, these fad diets like very low-carb plans don't work for sustainable weight loss [3].

That means there's a big chunk of Americans with a history of overeating and dieting, and that there's a good chance that many of us could use a course in satiety.

Pick Your Satiety Scale

With so many factors affecting how much we eat, it's important to start getting in touch with your own feelings of hunger and satiety. It's not impossible. It means checking in and rating your hunger and satisfaction by using a satiety scale.

If you're looking for an ultra-simple way to rate your satiety, use the "three Hs," Newgent says. Ask yourself if you're hungry, happy, or hurting. You should be hungry before you're satisfied, you're happy when you're satisfied, and you're hurting when you've eaten too much. The goal is to feel your hunger and get to a happy place, while avoiding hurting by eating too much [1].

That's a simplified version of a satiety scale. If you're looking for something with a little more nuance, try a ten-point scale. Before eating and while eating, ask yourself where you fall on a scale of one to ten [4].

- 0–2 Starving (your stomach might be eating itself!). You're very hungry and light-headed from lack of fuel.
- 3–4 Getting hungry, time to eat!
- 5 Neutral
- 6–7 Satisfied
- 8 Little too much, slow down next time!
- 9–10 Stuffed and sick. Some call it "Thanksgiving full"—eating that requires recovery, whether it's unbuttoning your belt and pants in front of the television or feeling the need to lie down while your food digests [4].

(http://www.bulimiahelp.org/tools/awareness/hunger-satiety-scale)

You don't want to get to nine or ten, but you also don't want to allow yourself to get to one or two. The hungrier you are when you start eating, the more likely you are to overeat [4].

Aim instead for middle ground. Your feelings of hunger and satiety should cycle between feeling slightly hungry and comfortably full throughout the day [4].

But there's one thing to keep in mind: It takes around ten minutes before your brain registers that you're at a five or six on the scale. That's why it's important to eat slowly and savor your food, put down your fork between bites, and to stop eating before you feel full. Otherwise, you'll go straight from hungry to overfull [4].

> *Instead of making each meal an inner battle, choose something healthy to eat, turn off the negative self-talk, and enjoy your food.*

Feeling Satisfied: Putting It into Practice

Knowing to stop eating when you're satisfied is one thing. Actually *doing* it is another. But there are ways to set yourself up for success.

Create Positive Inner Dialogue

It's hard to listen to your cues of satiety when you're constantly worried about what you're eating and cycling between overeating and deprivation. That leads to a constant dialogue in your head about food and weight [5].

It's normal to argue with yourself about what to eat at a restaurant, **but people with eating disorders have that type of inner conversation a hundred times a day**, says Amy Wood, PsyD. Instead of making each meal an inner battle, choose something healthy to eat, turn off the negative self-talk, and enjoy your food [5].

In fact, part of eating mindfully is understanding that there's no right or wrong way to eat, according to the Center for Mindful Eating. We hope that, by following our plan, you'll learn to approach eating with moderation [6].

Fuel Your Body Every Three to Four Hours

This goes back to not getting to a one on the satiety scale. Keeping your blood sugar level even by eating regularly throughout the day is more likely to lead to eating fewer calories by the time you turn in for the night, says H. Theresa Wright, MS, RD, LDN, founder of Renaissance Nutrition Center Inc. in East Norriton, PA [7].

Choose Whole Foods

Let's consider two lunch options:

A Snickers bar and a 12-ounce Coke for 423 calories [8].

Or three ounces of herbed chicken, mashed sweet potatoes with a pat of butter, five ounces of nonfat Greek yogurt with a half-cup of blueberries stirred in for 436 calories [8].

They're roughly the same number of calories, but which would make you feel more satisfied? You can bet it would be the chicken, potatoes, and fruit [7].

In general, foods that are high in nutrition and aren't processed are the most satisfying. You're more likely to find them in the produce, dairy, and meat sections of the supermarket than the inner aisles [7].

Take something like pop chips, a new snack that's being touted as a healthy alternative to traditional potato chips. Nineteen chips have only 120 calories and 4 grams of fat [9]. Sound like a good snack? It's probably not. "There's no satiety in this food," Wright says [7]. An apple and some nuts would be a better choice. While the chips may help in controlling cravings, they don't really satisfy hunger.

Make It a Balanced Meal

We might be sounding like a broken record, but it deserves to be mentioned again that eating a combination of protein, high-fiber carbohydrates (whole grains, vegetables, and fruit), and healthy fat will leave you more satisfied than eating only one type of food [4].

A breakfast of a vegetable omelet with a sliced orange will make you feel more satisfied than two pieces of toast and margarine. A turkey burger topped with vegetable slices on a whole-grain bun will be more filling than a macaroni salad.

Skip the Sugar Substitutes in Food

Studies on animals have found that we naturally associate sweet foods with high calories, so satiety will set in earlier after eating something very sweet [4].

Things change when you add sugar-free sweeteners to your food, such as saccharin (Sweet'N Low), aspartame (NutraSweet), sucralose (Splenda), and others. Researchers believe that in the long term, using calorie-free sweeteners interferes with your body's satiety cues [4].

Get Your Calories from Food, Not Drinks

Your brain may not register calories from liquids as well as it does from foods, so it's a good idea to skip sweet beverages like lemonade, sweetened tea, sports drinks, and soda in order to stay in touch with your feelings of satiety. One study found that when people were given 450 calories from soda or jelly beans, those who ate the jelly beans were more likely to eat fewer calories the rest of the day. When you do fill your cup with something sweet, drink those beverages in moderation. Arm yourself with the knowledge that, while soda tastes good, it is giving you calories without satisfying your hunger or giving you nutrition [4].

Always Use a Plate, and Always Sit Down at a Table

It's too easy to miss the feeling of satiety if you're eating out of the package while standing at the kitchen counter or out of a paper bag while driving your car. Make dining an event for three meals a day. Using a plate will help you visualize how much you have consumed. Sitting down and making food an event will encourage you to look at your portions and slow down your eating. You will find yourself refraining from snacking all day long or inhaling too many calories while mindlessly eating [4].

Focus on Eating

Once the food is on your plate, focus on your meal rather than looking at your iPhone, the TV, or the computer. You'll feel more satisfied after the meal, Newgent says [4]. Eating mindfully means choosing foods you like to eat that also nourish your body and allowing all of your senses to enjoy the food. Enjoy the essence of being human. You worked hard to purchase and/or prepare this food. Think about all the dynamics that have to happen to get that food on your table. You work because you need to eat to live. So savor your hard work! [6]

Make It a Small Plate

Take a look at your grandmother's or great-grandmother's china set, and compare the size of a dinner plate to the ones you have in your cupboard. Most likely, the older china is quite a bit smaller. Newer, larger plates reflect Americans' growing portion sizes.

If you have a bigger plate, you're more likely to fill it. (Kind of like the bigger your backpack, the more you'll put in it.) An example: when researchers gave a group of men and women potato chips on five different days, increasing the size of the bag each time, they ate significantly more from the bigger bags. Women consumed 18 percent more, while men chomped on 37 percent more chips [10].

The time to use a bigger plate is when you're filling your plate with mostly veggies, such as a big, fresh salad or grilled vegetables.

Sloooow Down

When you finish a meal in five minutes flat, your brain hasn't had a chance to catch up with your stomach and register satiety. A feeling of satisfaction usually comes about ten minutes after you've had enough, Newgent says. So be sure to put your fork down between bites and take it slow [4].

In the time it takes to feel satisfied, you could eat hundreds more calories if you're going too fast [4].

Relish the Tastes and Textures of Your Food

Eating is one of life's great pleasures. "It's a gift of the gods," Wright says. There's nothing wrong in really enjoying it. Sit back, listen to music while you eat, have a pleasant conversation with your family or friends, and eat as mindfully as you can [7].

Make It a Family Goal

Rather than being the only one eating from a small plate at the family dinner table, ask everyone to partake, Newgent suggests. Not only will you be more likely to keep it up when everyone else is, but your family will adopt healthier eating habits, too [4].

> *Your brain may not register calories from liquids as well as it does from foods, so it's a good idea to skip sweet beverages like lemonade, sweetened tea, sports drinks, and soda in order to stay in touch with your feelings of satiety.*

The bottom line: trust yourself. Dr. Wood has clients who are overweight and are able to diet and lose weight and then always gain the weight back. "I tell them not to be on a diet," she says. "Trust your intuition about when to eat and when to stop eating" [5].

Even if you fall off track 20 percent of the time, you can still be successful, she says [5].

Bottom Line

- Positive Self-Talk
- Whole Food Choices
- Savor the Flavor

A Sure Way to End up Unsatisfied: Go on a Fad Diet

"A diet is a short period of starvation that happens right before you gain twenty pounds," Wright says [7].

What Works for Me

Justin Doyle, worldwide training manager for Xerox Corp. in Rochester, NY

I've been battling my weight since my teens, and I've tried tons of fad diets over the years, from the cabbage soup diet, to low-carb diets to commercial diets. Some were highly successful and some weren't, but they all had one thing in common: Any weight I lost eventually made its way back on my frame.

I think the problem was that the weight loss happened inside a bubble. Each specific program assigned points or values to different foods, but once I stopped the diet and was eating in the real world again, I slid back into my old eating habits. Fad diets just weren't sustainable for me.

In April 2010, when I weighed 267 pounds, I decided I was going to lose weight again, and this time I was following my own plan.

I started with a personal trainer to kick-start my exercise. Then I tackled my diet. I found an online calorie-tracking tool and started plugging in everything I ate every day. I noticed right away that eating out was keeping me from losing weight. I used to think that getting a meal with grilled chicken was a healthy choice, but I failed to realize that the pasta and cream sauce the chicken came with had a deadly amount of fat and calories.

Early on, I went out to eat at the Cheesecake Factory and ordered chicken pot pie—and I probably washed it down with a couple of glasses of wine. I was shocked later to find out that the meal had close to 3,000 calories.

So, I started eating in a lot more often, and I even switched from stainless steel pans that required using butter and fat to keep food from sticking to nonstick pans. When I did go to a restaurant, I almost always looked up the nutrition information of their food first if it was available. Instead of getting dishes loaded with fat, I now order a steak salad with no dressing or dressing on the side.

Another factor was TV. I used to eat snacks like cheese and crackers, Chex Mix, and potato chips late at night while watching TV. I decided to cancel cable, in part to help me break that habit and also to save money. Instead of staying up late to watch the tube, I forced myself to go to bed. It took a while to stop craving those snacks in the evening, but after about a month of ignoring the urges they went away. It saved me hundreds of calories.

(continued)

(*continued*)

A little over a year later, I'm seventy-seven pounds lighter. I still keep track of calories and aim for 1,700 to 1,900 a day. I also exercise five or six days a week, and I'm running 5Ks and 10Ks. I have a goal to finish a half-marathon later this year. For me, the key was to tie weight loss to the real world. Once I did that, the weight dropped away.

When you sign up for a fad diet—the grapefruit diet, say, or a very low-carb diet—it's usually with high expectations. These diets promise big results in mere days or weeks. They also tend to rely on eating a special formulation of foods that supposedly leads to weight loss. Think of the blood type diet or a low-glycemic diet [11].

But the problem is that fad diets are hard to keep up, and they almost never help you keep the weight off in the long run [11].

The overriding theme of fad diets doesn't have to do with unlocking a secret formula to losing weight. They all drastically reduce the number of calories you eat [1, 11].

"You lose weight on fad diets because they're far too low in calories," Newgent says [1].

As a result, you don't get enough energy for your brain and muscles. You can't—and shouldn't—follow a fad diet for a lifetime. Fad diets also tend to be unbalanced. You don't get the proper mix of protein, carbohydrates, and fat, Newgent says [1].

Also, when you restrict your calorie intake that severely, you set yourself up for a serious rebound. "The body is programmed for survival," Wright says [7].

When cavemen and cavewomen roamed the earth, they ate a lot when food was available in the summer and lived on stored fat in the winter. That means your body was designed to survive a fad diet without dropping much weight—or by dropping weight and putting it on again quickly [7].

When you starve your body, your metabolism drops to conserve calories. And when you go off a very low-calorie diet, you'll want to eat more and more to replace the fat stores you just lost, Wright says. It's all too easy to lose less weight than you wanted and then pack it on again once you stop the diet [7].

The meal plan in this book is not a fad diet; it's a healthy way of eating that will lead to weight loss. But it's easy to fall for the promises of a fad diet. Here are five signs you're on a fad diet:

- You expect to lose more than one or two pounds a week.
- Your choices in food are limited, and the diet isn't balanced.

- The diet is expensive and requires you to buy products to lose weight.
- The diet oversimplifies medical research.
- It sounds too good to be true [11].

Still Feeling Out of Control?

"The best thing I can do to make a compulsive eater binge is to get her good and hungry," says Wright. Normal eaters will go overboard when they let themselves get too hungry, but someone with a food addiction has a much stronger reaction, she says [7].

If you're continually eating past the point of feeling full, there is help. Therapy is an option, or you can go to a place and get support from people who know exactly what you're going through: an Overeaters Anonymous (OA) meeting [7].

"Overeaters Anonymous is a powerful force," says Wright. "It helps you put down the food and embark on a journey of emotional and spiritual growth" [7].

If the only thing you know about OA is from what you've seen on the CBS sitcom "Mike and Molly," you might think that it's for people who are very overweight or obese. It is, but it's also for people who are a little overweight or not overweight at all. In fact, its 54,000 members range from being morbidly obese to underweight [12, 13].

But they all have one thing in common: They want to stop eating compulsively. Food is more than a physiological feeling and need for them [13].

The meetings are open to anyone who feels out of control with their eating, says Naomi Lippel, managing director of OA Inc., in Rio Rancho, N.M. An unhealthy relationship with food can affect you physically, emotionally, and spiritually. OA meetings work on changing that [13].

The group uses a twelve-step program to deal with compulsive eating. OA also is a place where you can find support from people who know exactly what you're going through, and you'll have a sponsor to guide you [12].

Although it's a spiritual program, it's nondenominational. It's also free of charge. The organization is supported through members' voluntary contributions, Lippel says [12].

When people finally acknowledge that they need something outside of themselves to recover from compulsive eating, OA is there for them [12]. All you have to do is find a meeting near you. There are about 6,500 OA meetings being held in more than seventy-five countries (http://www.oa.org/) [13].

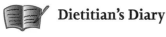 **Dietitian's Diary**

Hydration

Hydration is the key to allowing your body to give you proper hunger signals, while also preventing headaches, detoxifying metabolic by-products, and aiding post workout rejuvenation and healing. Proper hydration is important because our bodies are more than half water. Water transports nutrients, regulates our body temperature, aids in digestion, and gets rid of waste.

Your Body's Needs

To avoid being thirsty, drink eight to ten cups of non alcoholic, caffeine-free fluid a day. This equals about two liters of fluid. For those refilling 16-ounce water bottles, this is five bottles a day. Water is the quickest and cheapest way to hydrate, but other fluids count too. Milk, juice, and water in fruits and vegetables all contribute to your daily fluid intake. Water, however, is the only natural, calorie-free way to hydrate. (See Chapter 13 for ideas for adding flavor without artificial sweeteners and keeping it low in calories.)

Dehydration can mimic the feeling of hunger. As you learn to recognize the hunger signals your body is sending you, think about how much fluid you have had to drink during the day. There are times in our days when it is more difficult to drink enough fluids because of our jobs or schedule.

Seasonal changes can make it more difficult to get enough fluids. Our desire to drink cold water in the winter and in the summer fluctuates. If you are in the Midwest, it may be easy to get enough water in the winter by warming up with your hot tea, but it is also dehydrating you. In the summer in the Southwest it is easy to get enough water because of the heat. But use eight to ten cups as a guide for your needs all year 'round.

If you're not sure whether you're hungry or thirsty, look back at how much fluid you have consumed in the day. Drink a glass of water and wait a few minutes. This may help your body adjust and help you figure out if you are hungry or thirsty. And when you are eating a meal, choose a calorie-free or low-calorie beverage to enjoy with your meal. About three-quarters of our daily fluid consumption happens while we are eating.

Recipes

CAJUN JAMBALAYA   Serves: 6

3 tablespoons garlic, minced
2 celery stalks, chopped
1 red bell pepper, chopped
½ cup yellow onion, chopped
2 tablespoons canola oil

1 tablespoon liquid smoke
3 cups vegetable broth
2 cups brown rice
1 teaspoon chili sauce, hot sauce
3 bay leaves
1 15 oz. can chopped tomatoes
1 tablespoon Cajun Spice (recipe below)
12 medium shrimp, peeled, deveined, and cut in half
2 chicken sausages, apple flavored, sliced into half circles

Directions:

1. Sauté garlic, celery, pepper, and onion in canola oil.

2. Add remaining ingredients (except shrimp and sausage).

3. Bring to a boil.

4. Turn down heat and simmer for 30 minutes or until rice is cooked through.

5. Add shrimp and sausage and cook until shrimp has turned pink.

6. Serve warm.

Pre Servings: 390 calories, 8.2 g fat, 61 g carbohydrate, 1.9 g fiber, 18.3 g protein.

CAJUN SPICE

1 teaspoon sea salt
Zest of half a lemon
2½ tablespoons paprika
2 tablespoons garlic powder
1 tablespoon onion powder
½ tablespoon cayenne pepper
1 ½ tablespoons dried oregano
1 tablespoon thyme

FRESH FRUIT GRANOLA   Serves: 1

½ cup granola, low fat
½ cup blueberries
½ cup Greek yogurt
2 tablespoons flaxseed meal

Directions:

1. Mix all together and serve.

Per serving: 305 calories, 5.2 g fat, 55 g carbohydrate, 5.1 g fiber, 9.7 g protein.

FIGGY QUINOA PUDDING   **Serves: 5**

1 cup quinoa
1 ½ cups soy milk, plain, light
4 tablespoons brandy extract
6 dried figs, chopped

Directions:

1. Combine 1½ cup of soy milk and 1 cup rinsed quinoa.

2. Bring to a boil.

3. Turn down heat and simmer for 15 minutes.

4. Remove from heat.

5. Let sit 15 minutes.

6. Stir in brandy extract and dried figs.

TIP

Store extra in the refrigerator and reheat for the next day breakfast or a sweet snack.

Per serving: 181 calories, 2.6 g fat, 33 g carbohydrate, 2.2 g fiber, 6.4 g protein.

Throwing Exercise into the Mix

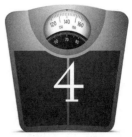

Learn How Exercise Can Help You Burn Off the 3,500 Calories Stored in Every Pound of Fat and Keep Hunger in Check by Suppressing Your Appetite

You can't lose weight without changing the way you eat, but there's more to weight loss than what you put in your mouth. An essential part of losing weight is working up a sweat.

A great workout can burn 500 to 1,000 calories, and that can go a long way toward helping you chip away at the 3,500 calories in every pound of fat [1, 2].

What's more, studies have found that a heart-pumping aerobic workout can release hormones that actually suppress your hunger, making it even easier to stick to a weight-loss plan [3, 4].

But unfortunately in today's world, exercise doesn't happen on its own—certainly not during the typical workday when we're sitting on desk chairs or having business lunches. "Nothing in our natural existence makes us breathe hard," says Christina Walman, a group fitness instructor in Santa Barbara, C.A. "We have to be intentional about pushing up our heart rates" [5].

But if personal trainers had a dollar for every person they've heard say they don't like exercise, well, you know how rich they would be. The truth is that exercise is nonnegotiable. And no matter how much you think you're going to hate it, your body was meant to move and will reward you when you give it what it wants [2, 5].

> Researchers have looked at the effect exercise has on hormones that influence hunger, and several studies have found that exercise may suppress hunger hours or even days after finishing a workout.

Why You Can't Skip Working Out

Perhaps the most compelling reason to exercise is this: People who have lost weight and kept it off long term say that exercise is a big part of their success [6].

The National Weight Control Registry has studied five thousand people who have lost weight and kept it off. Among them, 94 percent say they increased their physical activity to lose weight. Most often, walking was their form of exercise. And in order to keep the weight off, 90 percent say they exercise about an hour a day [6].

But there are many more reasons to work out.

It Can Suppress Your Appetite

Researchers have looked at the effect exercise has on hormones that influence hunger, and several studies have found that exercise may suppress hunger hours or even days after finishing a workout [3].

In one study, eleven male students participated in three 8-hour sessions with researchers. In the first session, they ran on a treadmill for sixty minutes and rested for seven hours. In the second session, they lifted weights for ninety minutes and rested the remainder of the time. And in the third session, they didn't exercise at all. The researchers asked them about their hunger levels, gave them two meals, and measured levels of ghrelin and peptide YY, two hormones that help to regulate appetite [3, 4].

The study found that working out on the treadmill led to hormone changes that suppressed their appetite. Although they reported feeling less hungry after lifting weights, their hormone levels after strength training were mixed, and the study authors said they're still not sure if it lowers appetite [3].

Moderate exercise is also known to make people more sensitive to insulin, which means their bodies do a better job of keeping their blood sugar levels stable. When your blood sugar levels are more stable, you'll avoid spikes and steep drops in blood sugar that can make you hungry [7].

You'll Have More Energy Than You Thought You Had

People who are sedentary report having loads more energy when they start exercising. In one study of thirty-six people who complained of being tired, working out at a low or moderate intensity boosted their energy by 20 percent. They also reported a 65 percent decline in fatigue [8, 9].

It only takes about a week. By your second week of exercising, you'll be stronger, have more endurance, and feel more energized than you did before you started working out, says Shaun A. Zetlin, a certified master trainer in the New York City metro area [2].

Exercise Boosts Your Mood and Lowers Your Stress Level

Exercise is an incredible stress reliever. "I can be an anxious person sometimes, and for me, exercise is the most amazing remedy," Zetlin says. He says he has even trained a few therapists who told him they tell their patients to try exercise before medication [2].

In fact, researchers who have analyzed dozens of studies have found that exercise can act as a drug to relieve depression and anxiety [10].

If you've ever picked up a cookie or swung into a fast food drive-thru when you were stressed or feeling depressed, you know how important stress relief can be in changing your eating habits.

You'll Gain Loads of Confidence

When you finish that first mile or first 5K, or become strong enough to do push-ups on your toes instead of your knees, or make it to the top of the hill without stopping for a rest, or climb the stairs at work without becoming winded, your confidence level will skyrocket. And that confidence will spread to every area of your life [5].

"Everybody I know—client or not—who takes up and sustains an exercise program gains positive self-esteem," Walman says. When you start doing something you know you should be doing—like exercising—you naturally start doing other things you know you should be doing, whether it's sticking to an eating plan or advancing your career [5].

Even when you don't lose weight right away, exercise will make you feel great in your skin and, as an added bonus, your clothes will fit better [11].

Because You *Are* an Athlete

Reset your identity from being someone who thinks you don't like exercise or isn't very good at exercise to being an athlete, because everyone—*everyone*—has an inner athlete, Walman says. When you find the right activity that works for you, you'll excel at it, and you'll want to do it every day [5].

For some people, running makes them feel elated. For others, it's bike riding or swimming or dancing or rowing or martial arts. "Just because a particular athletic activity isn't your thing doesn't mean you're disqualified as an athlete," Walman says. "We're businesspeople, we're spouses, we're parents, and we're athletes" [5].

Still dubious? Everyone has at least one exercise they like, Zetlin says. And once you find something you love, you'll be amazed at what you can do. "There are a lot of people out there who weren't athletes in high school but have surprised themselves by what they can do physically," he says [2]. Odds are, you don't know how strong and resilient your body is, so it's time to find out.

How Much Do You Need to Do?

To lose weight and maintain weight loss, research says you need to work out for 275 minutes a week. That's fifty-five minutes, five days a week or forty-five minutes, six days a week [12].

If that sounds discouraging, start by doing what you can. "People get this idea that if they can't do it all they should just forget it," says Walman. But when you make the smallest movement in the right direction, it becomes easier and easier [5].

If all you can do are abdominal crunches or push-ups for sixty seconds, then do it. That might lead to a sixty-second wall squat, which might lead to a brisk walk, and before you know it, you're working up a sweat [5].

Even if your workout is short right now (you can put in ten minutes on the treadmill, let's say), set a goal of adding one or two minutes to each exercise session. That's how you increase your confidence and workout time simultaneously [11].

Research has also found that exercising for just ten minutes three times a day or fifteen minutes twice a day is as effective as one thirty-minute workout. In one study of forty-eight overweight female college students, researchers divided them into four groups: one that exercised for thirty minutes, one that exercised for ten minutes three times a day, one that exercised for fifteen minutes twice a day, and one that didn't exercise at all. After twelve weeks, the researchers found that shorter workouts two or three times a day had the same effect on weight loss and fitness levels as exercising for thirty minutes straight [13].

Get Moving: Find Your Exercise Personality

If you're new to exercise, start in your comfort zone. Maybe it's walking or a beginner's class at the gym [5].

And once you're more comfortable moving your body, challenge yourself. It may mean hiring a personal trainer, signing up for a more advanced class, or committing to a 5K walk or run [5].

This is a good rule-of-thumb: Work out at between 55 percent and 85 percent of your maximum ability, says Zetlin. Someone on the elliptical trainer at the gym who is not sweating and can read a book is working out at about 55 percent, he says. But someone who's working hard and sweating but can still give you a smile is at about 85 percent. The goal is to get to 85 percent—you're working hard but you're not collapsing [2].

Also, aim for an exercise routine that combines strength training, such as lifting weights, with aerobic exercise, such as walking or aerobics [2]. That's the best strategy for weight loss, toning, and your overall health [11].

So, what are you going to do? Walking, jogging, Pilates, yoga, cycling, and kickboxing are options that may already be on your radar screen. The American Council on Exercise also has an online exercise library with detailed information on strength exercises you can do on your own [14].

If those activities still don't sound appealing, here's a list of ways to get your heart pumping that you may not have thought of.

- Dance classes, such as Zumba, modern dance, hip hop, ballet, ballroom, or salsa
- Martial arts
- Tai chi
- Rowing or sailing clubs
- Outdoor classes, such as boot camp
- Downhill or cross-country skiing
- Ice skating
- Roller skating or roller derby
- Rock climbing gyms
- Hiking
- Swimming or water aerobics
- Sports, such as basketball, football, soccer, softball, volleyball, or hockey

Planning Your Meals Around Exercise

The key to losing weight while exercising is to plan your meals and snacks around your workouts, says Zetlin. If you don't, you could set yourself up to be too tired during a workout, or you could become so ravenously hungry afterward that you blow your eating plan.

What Works for Me

Ellen Stenzel, a high school Spanish teacher in Rochester, N.Y.

I started working out in college, about fifteen years ago. Although I felt a little discouraged at first because I tired out so quickly, it didn't take long before I started really enjoying it. Seeing my body gain muscle tone, lose fat, and having people compliment me on the way I looked kept me going.

About four years ago, I lost thirty pounds through diet and exercise, and exercise has certainly helped me keep it off since then. I work out for forty to sixty

(continued)

(*continued*)

minutes about four or five days a week on an elliptical trainer, stationary bike, or on the treadmill at the gym. I also walk, jog, and do hills and sprints outside of the gym, and I took a six-week boot camp class last summer. On top of that, I take classes at a yoga studio.

I continue to exercise, mostly for the feeling of exhilaration that comes midway through and after a workout. Exercise also gives me time to meditate or get rid of anger in a constructive way.

The benefits definitely spill over into other aspects of my life. When I exercise regularly, I adopt the attitude that I need to "fuel the machine," and I make healthier food choices and drink more water. Because I'm hungry after a workout, I keep a 100-calorie pack of almonds and a piece of fruit in the car, or I have a protein shake on the way home from the gym.

And remember that exercising doesn't give you license to indulge in a donut or something else that's going to undermine your weight loss efforts [2]. When you work out really hard at the gym, remind yourself that you don't want to interfere with your progress with a beer or a piece of cake [11]. Here's what to do:

An Hour or Two Before Your Workout

Eat a light meal or snack. If you head to the gym straight from work, make sure you have a snack that's a combination of protein and carbohydrates about an hour before you leave [2].

If you're an early morning exerciser, eat something small as soon as you wake up so you'll have the energy for a great workout [2].

Within an Hour After Finishing Your Workout

Have a healthy meal waiting for you at home, or pack a healthy snack in your car to hold you over until you can eat a meal [2].

Physical Activity Is Your Friend

It's time to stop procrastinating and weave an exercise plan into your life. It will burn calories, boost physical strength and confidence, and be an ally in your fight against that ever-present nemesis: **hunger**.

 A good rule of thumb: Work out at between 55 percent and 85 percent of your maximum ability.

Exercise Personality Quiz

Zetlin offers the following Exercise Personality Quiz. Try it—it's fun!

1. The thought of going to the gym before or after work makes you feel:
   A. Anxious
   B. Thrilled
   C. Upset
   D. Happy

2. How knowledgeable do you feel when it comes to strength and cardio-vascular training?
   A. Lost
   B. Excited
   C. Frustrated
   D. Confident

3. When performing a cardiovascular workout on the treadmill, elliptical, or stationary bike, how do you feel?
   A. Apprehensive
   B. Motivated
   C. Bored
   D. Comfortable

4. Your friend asks you to work out with him or her at your local gym. What do you feel?
   A. Nervous
   B. Energized
   C. Distraught
   D. Ecstatic

5. The thought of keeping a journal and writing down your progress while working out creates an emotion of:
   A. Dread
   B. Exhilaration
   C. Annoyance
   D. Contentment

6. The notion of missing a workout during the week makes you feel:
   A. Relieved
   B. Distressed
   C. Satisfied
   D. Disappointed

7. Finding the time in your current schedule to work out creates a sensation of:
   A. Concern
   B. Freedom
   C. Stress
   D. Bliss

8. After exercising, you usually feel:
   A. Defeated
   B. Hyper
   C. Miserable
   D. Cheerful

If you answered "A" for most of these questions, your Exercise Personality is:
Fearful
The thought of working out and going to the gym seems scary to you. However, try to change your mindset by exercising in the privacy of your own home. Next, enlist a trusted family member or friend to show you some beginner movements at the gym. Exercising doesn't have to be scary; it be very empowering if you are open to it.

If you answered "B" for most of these questions, your Exercise Personality is:
Manic
Being manic isn't necessarily a negative personality trait, yet it is crucial to understand why working out is so important to you. Anyone who exercises consistently deserves an ovation. But missing a workout shouldn't leave you devastated. Bravo for staying committed to exercise, but give yourself a much-needed break by skipping your workout a few times a week, and your muscles will tone faster!

If you answered "C" for most of these questions, your Exercise Personality is:
Discouraged
It's quite normal to feel discouraged when starting an exercise program or if you have been working out for years without seeing the desired results. It might be time to hire a fitness professional to help you reach your fitness goals faster than you would on your own. Work on staying positive and committed.

If you answered "D" for most of these questions your Exercise Personality is:
Joyful
You have a healthy relationship with working out and enjoy exercise to its fullest. Working out makes you feel carefree and blissful, which, in its purity, is what it's supposed to do! You can help keep that joy in your workouts by

varying your workout every few months. When you change your routine, be sure to choose exercises that make you feel happy, but are still challenging.

Dietitian's Diary

Food and Exercise

Before your workout you will want a snack that is low in fat and fiber for optimal digestion. A snack with protein and carbohydrates is a great choice. Protein helps repair and build muscles used in exercise and may help with postworkout soreness.

Carbohydrates help boost your energy level in order to have a great workout. Try something like a smoothie or fruit and a piece of low-fat cheese. See the charts below and choose one item each from the protein and carbohydrate charts.

After your workout you will want to eat a balanced meal or snack to replenish what is lost during exercise. You'll need fluids and electrolytes, including sodium and potassium, carbohydrates, and protein. Fluids and electrolytes are necessary to replenish what your body lost during exercise through sweat. If you plan to eat a meal right away, make sure to drink plenty of nonalcoholic fluids.

If you don't plan to eat a meal for more than an hour after exercising, have a small snack. Sodium and potassium will come naturally from the protein and carbohydrate items, with carbohydrates yielding more potassium. Choose one item from each of the snack grids below.

Carbohydrates High in Potassium	Serving Size	Calories
Apricots	2 raw or 5 dry	34
Banana	1 medium	105
Bran muffin	2 ounces (1 small)	153
Cantaloupe	½ cup	39
Dates	5 each	120
Dried figs	2	42
Granola with fruit and nuts	¼ cup	140
Honeydew melon	½ cup	41
Kiwi	1 medium	46
Mango	1	135
Nectarine or orange	1 medium	62
Pear	1 medium	96

(Continued)

Carbohydrates High in Potassium	Serving Size	Calories
Papaya	½ medium fruit	59
Pomegranate seeds	½ cup	72
Prunes	5	101
Raisins	¼ cup	123
Orange juice	½ cup	56
Grapefruit juice	½ cup	45
Prune juice	½ cup	90
Pomegranate juice	½ cup	79

Protein	Serving Size	Calories
Mozzarella cheese, part skim	1 ounce	71
Low-fat cottage cheese	½ cup	82
Hard-boiled egg, no yolk	1 large egg	17
Sliced turkey	1 ounce (about 1 slice)	29
Extra lean ham	1 ounce (about 1 slice)	31
Fat-free milk	8 ounces (1 cup)	91
Plain soy milk	8 ounces (1 cup)	100
Peanut butter	1 tablespoon	94
Roasted pumpkin seeds	1 ounce (85 seeds)	126
Roasted sunflower seeds	½ ounce (⅛ cup)	83
Yogurt	6 ounces	95

Recipes

QUICK PRE- OR POST-EXERCISE SMOOTHIE   Serves: 2

2 tablespoons peanut butter
2 cups skim or soy milk
1 large banana

Mix together in a blender or food processor.
Or, build your own smoothies using the grid below.

SMOOTHIE GRID   Serves: 2

Liquid		Fruit and Vegetables	Fat and More Fiber
Protein	**Carbohydrate**	**Carbohydrate**	
Tofu, soft, ½ cup	100% juice, ⅓ cup	1 cup frozen fruit, any kind	Nut Butter—2 Teaspoons
Soy milk, light and plain, 1 cup	Other juice, ½ cup	1 cup canned fruit, drained and rinsed	Flaxseed Meal—4 Tablespoons
Soy milk, chocolate and light, 1 cup		1 cup fresh fruit, with peel or without peel	
1% milk, 1 cup		1 cup green leafy vegetable, kale or spinach	
Skim milk, 1 cup			
Yogurt, plain— ⅔ cup			
Yogurt, Greek— ⅔ cup			

1. Combine a total of 1½ cups liquid (if juice is used, only one serving) in a blender or food processor.

2. Add a total of 2 servings fruit and/or vegetables.

3. Combine 1–2 servings of nut butter and/or flaxseed.

TIP

For kale, remove rib in center of leaf before blending.

And, to go with your smoothie, build a satisfying wrap as a quick post-exercise meal.

SATISFACTION SOLUTION WRAP GRID   Serves: 1

Wrap	Protein 1–2 Servings	Vegetables, 1 Cup	Flavor
• flatbread	Beans, ½ cup	Salad greens	Vinegars
• whole wheat tortilla	Bean spread/dip, ½ cup	Corn	• Balsamic, white and red
• whole gain tortilla	Leftover meat, 1 ounce	Beets	• Rice vinegar
	Lunch meat, 1 ounce	Broccoli	• Apple cider vinegar
	Cheese, 1 ounce	Carrots	Juice
		Celery	• Lime juice
		Cucumber	• Lemon juice
		Onion	• Orange juice
		Jicama	• Pineapple juice
		Mushrooms	• Grapefruit juice
		Bell peppers	• Mayonnaise/ Vegenaise, 1 tablespoon or less
		Tomatoes	
		Squash	
		Radishes	
		Water chestnuts	

1. Combine protein, vegetable, and flavor ingredients.
2. Place mixture in wrap and enjoy!

Revving Up for Weight Loss

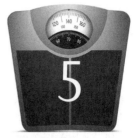

Learn How to Get Ready for Successful Weight Loss

We're hoping you're getting pumped for some serious weight loss by now. But before you dive into the eating plan our dietitian created for you in Part Two, it's time to get truly ready for success.

There are two things that will be crucial to losing weight while staying satisfied: planning your meals and always leaving the house prepared.

Step One: Plan Your Meals

A big part of eating healthy and staying satisfied throughout the day is about planning. We know that everyone is busy. People are working long hours and juggling multiple responsibilities, and that tends to be why they say they don't have time to cook.

Here's the truth: It takes less time than you think to shop for and prepare meals at home. "We think it's a lot of work when it's really not," H. Theresa Wright of the Renaissance Nutrition Center Inc. says. "We are making it too hard on ourselves."

And when you do take the time to plan and cook your own meals, you're saving yourself tons of calories (compared to eating out), and you're preparing meals that are filled with nutrients that keep you healthy, protect you from disease, and help you feel satisfied. Look at it as preventative medicine.

It's also cheaper. Wright had a client who spent between $350 to $500 a month on mocha lattes and diet sodas—food that fills you up on empty calories and makes your body crave more food.

Cutting out those expensive drinks that aren't adding anything to your diet and focusing on healthy meals will help you feel fuller while saving money. Save those extra dollars to buy yourself some new clothes in a smaller size.

Food Shop Once a Week

Wright recommends planning your meals for the week and buying the food you need in one shopping trip. That means you're prepared with a full week of healthy meals, and you won't have to return to the store later in the week to be tempted by food that will blow your eating plan.

This is how she makes one trip to buy fruits and vegetables that last the week:

- Buy berries that are ready to eat today and tomorrow, peaches and nectarines for the next two days, apples and oranges that will stay fresh in the fridge for a week or two, and a pineapple that won't be ripe for four or five days.

- Buy enough fresh greens and vegetables to last three or four days, and rely on frozen steam-in-the-bag veggies for the rest of the week. If you don't have the time to chop vegetables, buy some bags of cut-up vegetables, or choose ones you like from the salad bar at the store.

Stock Up on Healthy, Convenient Meals

While you're at the store, it's a good idea to get a few healthy microwave meals to have on hand if you find yourself without a preplanned lunch or dinner. Buy the good ones: Amy's Kitchen organic meals, CedarLane, Ethnic Gourmet, and Tandoor Chef. "Buy a dozen so you can come home from work and throw one in the microwave," Wright says. Add a fruit and a vegetable to the meal to make it a Satisfaction Solution meal.

Shop Produce Stands

If you do run out of produce before the week is out, go to a produce stand instead of the supermarket, Wright recommends. You'll get exactly what you need for satisfying meals without having to stare down the candy bars by the checkout counter.

Designate a Cooking Day

People think it takes a lot of time and work to plan out meals and prepare them for the week, but it really doesn't. "It takes two to three hours, especially if you get the kids involved in washing and chopping produce," Wright says. "It's not as big of a deal as we imagine."

Prepare enough chicken to eat for that day's dinner, and season and cook the rest in a skillet, on the grill, or in the oven. Then put individual servings in Ziploc bags and freeze them for later in the week.

Make Mondays Meatless

Meatless Mondays are a new trend, and everybody's doing it. You should, too. This is a way to get in some healthy protein sources without turning to the usuals: chicken, beef, pork, or turkey. If you'll be following the food plan in Part II of this book, Meatless Mondays will be built right into your eating plan. You'll save money and time; no more waiting for meat to thaw or cook.

Rethink Dinner

Dinner doesn't always have to be a piece of meat with veggies and a starch. A wonderfully satisfying meal can be a baked potato topped with cottage or ricotta cheese, garlic, parmesan cheese, and steamed vegetables such as broccoli, carrots, and snow peas, Wright says.

Reuse Leftovers

Spread a healthy meal over a few dinners by freezing your leftovers in freezer-safe containers or bags and enjoying them a few days later. Put the food in the freezer within three to four days and be sure to thaw the foods safely in the refrigerator, microwave, or cold water. Cooked meat, soups, stews, and casseroles can be frozen for up to two to three months while maintaining their quality [1].

Step Two: Always Leave the House Prepared

If you're trying to lose weight, you might feel as if you shouldn't be caught with food shoved in your briefcase or purse. But that's exactly what you *should* do. Take these approaches when you're leaving the house, and you won't be caught hungry without a healthy meal.

Eat Before You Leave

Remember that it's normal to get hungry every three to four hours. If you're going to be out of the house for several hours and you're not planning to eat a meal while you're out, have a satisfying snack before you leave [2].

"I usually eat before I go out," says Melissa Paris, a certified nutritionist, certified personal trainer, and owner of Melissa Paris Fitness in New York City. When she has an event to attend in the evenings, she might have a yogurt with flaxseeds before she leaves so she doesn't even think about the food table while she's out. This healthy pre-snack helps her avoid high-calorie delights. And chances are her hosts never notice [2].

Keep Healthy Snacks with You on the Go

Paris also says she doesn't leave the house without a healthy snack with her, such as trail mix, a high-fiber bar, or an apple and two tablespoons of almond butter in a small container [2].

Road Trip? Pack a Cooler

If you're going to be in the car, pack a cooler with healthy wraps or sandwiches and vegetables to dip into hummus, such as celery and carrots, rather than stopping to eat out [2]. For a snack high in fiber, pack the Satisfaction Solution Black Bean Dip in your cooler (see recipe on page 197).

Stick with What You Know

When you do have to eat in a place that you're not familiar with, such as an airport or another country, choose foods that you already know well, Paris suggests. Opt for salads with vinaigrette dressing and plenty of fruits and vegetables while steering away from a lot of rich cheeses and desserts [2].

Stay Strong

Before you use being away from home as an excuse to dive into a greasy burger and fries, ask yourself how you're going to feel after eating something that's way off your food plan. Instead, order a hamburger and eat half of it, and order a side of broccoli instead of fries, Paris recommends [2].

Eat Out Smart

Gone are the days when families indulged in a restaurant meal only on special occasions, like a birthday. Half of the money Americans spend on food today is at restaurants or food stands, according to the Rudd Center for Food Policy and Obesity at Yale University [3].

For many Americans, one-third of their calories come from fast-food restaurants or food vendors, and it's no coincidence that as people eat out more, the incidence of obesity, diabetes, and heart disease rises [3].

What's wrong with taking a day off from cooking? The problem is, food that you eat out can be so packed with fat and calories that it's hard even for nutritionists to estimate how many calories it contains [3].

For example, gulping a venti (24-ounce) strawberry and crème frappuccino at Starbucks will give you a shocking 750 calories, according to the Center for Science in the Public Interest (CSPI). An innocent-looking slice of carrot cake at the Cheesecake Factory delivers an outrageous 1,560 calories.

Snack on a large popcorn with butter topping at the movie theater and you'll be munching more than 1,600 calories [4].

The kicker: None of these foods are even meals. They're what you eat after a meal or between meals. And even if you shared them with another person, you're probably getting quite a bit more calories than you bargained for.

There's a push by groups like the Rudd Center and CSPI to require restaurants to post nutrition information in a place where consumers can easily find it, and the federal government recently granted their wish. A new FDA regulation put in place on June 30, 2012 states that chain restaurants must provide easy-to-find nutrition information about their food [5]. If you see how much damage the food can do if not enjoyed in moderation, you might just lose your appetite for that food. Right now, nutrition information is available for about half of the chain restaurants out there, but in many cases it takes some work by you to track it down [3].

It's always better to cook your meals at home because you'll have control over the quality of the ingredients and how much fat and calories you consume, but we know you're going to eat out. Eating out is a nice indulgence that plenty of us look forward to doing. Research shows that, on average, Americans eat four meals away from home a week [4].

You're planning the meals you eat at home. Now it's time to plan for when you're out of the house.

Get the Nutrition Information

You can't just walk into a restaurant blind. Restaurant food can have more calories than you might imagine. Take the Farmhouse Cheeseburger at the Cheesecake Factory. It's loaded with 1,503 calories, 36 grams of fat, and 3,210 milligrams of sodium. If you also eat the fries on the plate, you'll bump up your calorie intake to 1,990! This is more calories than most people should eat in an entire day [5]!

The moral of the story? Look up the nutrition information on the restaurant's website or on a website like CalorieKing.com before you go, so you know what you're getting yourself into when you place your order. Plus, seek out the healthy options listed on some chain restaurants' website and menus.

Have a Snack Before You Go

It might seem counterintuitive, but it's good to eat before you go to a restaurant if you think you'll be starving by the time you sit down to eat. The intense food smells of some restaurants are too much to handle when you have a growling stomach, and that means you may scarf down hundreds—even thousands—of calories before you know it. Grab a banana or some carrots to help curb the desire to inhale fat-packed appetizers.

Go Easy on the Extras

It's a real bummer when you're stuffed before your meal even arrives because of the bread, salad, chips, appetizers, or drinks you consumed before your order arrived. Rather than indulging in the bread, an appetizer, wine, and dessert, pick and choose what you really want. Choosing a glass of wine, your meal, and a few bites of dessert that you share with everyone at the table can help you feel satisfied without being overstuffed.

Stick with Your Usual Healthy Meals

Once you've done research on a meal and you know it fits into your healthy eating plan, keep ordering it. People who tend to eat the same foods also tend to be the most successful at weight loss. And, when the point comes that you're ready for a change, you'll know how to research healthy options [6].

Ask for Half

You've probably heard this advice before: Ask your server to bring just half of your meal and pack the other half to go so you're not tempted to finish everything on your plate.

Personalize Your Meal

If the meal comes with fried chicken, ask for grilled. If the pasta usually comes swimming in a cheesy sauce, ask for no sauce or sauce on the side. When you order a salad, ask for the dressing on the side. If the meal comes with a side of fries, ask for a side of veggies instead.

Keep Your Satiety Scale Handy

This is the perfect time to practice listening to your satiety cues. Keep a copy of your satiety scale in your pocket or your purse, and place it on the table or discreetly in your lap as a reminder that you need to stay in touch with how full you're feeling throughout the meal.

Slow Down and Sit Down

Slow down your pace. This will help you enjoy your meal and company. Sometimes we feel pressured to eat faster when the waiter keeps coming by. But relax; this is your time to get energized and rejuvenated with a healthy meal and fluids.

If you are on the go, try your best to sit down at a table to eat your meal, rather than making the meal to-go. Eating mindlessly in the car is not only dangerous, but it can also cause you to eat past your satisfaction point.

Plan an Activity for After Dinner

Rather than going home and retiring in front of the television, try burning off some of those calories by going dancing or taking a long walk on the city streets or through a park.

Quiz: What'll You Have?

Although the calorie counts at some eateries may seem dismal to someone embarking on a weight-loss journey, smart ordering can keep you on track. Do you know which option is your best bet?

1. **You're at a donut shop. What are you ordering?**
   A. An old-fashioned cake donut
   B. A croissant sandwich with egg
   C. An egg white sandwich

   Answer: The egg white sandwich with veggies at Dunkin' Donuts is a good option at 280 calories and 10 grams of fat—better than an egg croissant sandwich at 480 calories and 29 grams of fat. Without the frosting, jelly, or sprinkles, you would think the plain old cake donut wouldn't be quite so bad, but it's 320 calories and 22 grams of fat. How satisfied do you think you'll feel after eating it? Odds are, not very satisfied [7].

2. **You're at a coffee shop. What are you ordering?**
   A. A coffee with skim milk
   B. A caffè latte
   C. A caffè mocha

   Answer: Assuming it's not a substitute for a nutritious meal, a 12-ounce coffee is your best option. Black, it's only 5 calories, but if you add non-fat milk it's only about 18 calories. A tall caffè latte with whole milk at Starbucks, on the other hand, carries with it 180 calories and 9 grams of fat. A caffè mocha with whole milk and whipped cream delivers 290 calories and 15 grams of fat [8].

3. **You're at a fast food joint for breakfast. What are you ordering?**
   A. Platter of pancakes, syrup, scrambled eggs, a biscuit, sausage, and hash browns

B. Oatmeal and fruit
C. An egg, cheese, and sausage sandwich

Answer: You probably guessed that a platter of breakfast food from a fast-food restaurant isn't a good idea. Burger King's Ultimate Breakfast Platter comes in at a heart-stopping 1,310 calories and 72 grams of fat. A breakfast sandwich on a muffin pales in comparison, at 410 calories and 26 grams of fat. Your best breakfast choice: look for a place that has fruit and oatmeal, such as McDonald's or Starbucks. You'll get a satisfying breakfast for 290 calories and 4.5 grams of fat, with 5 grams of fiber to boot [9, 10].

4. **You're at the "Golden Arches" at lunchtime. What are you ordering?**
   A. A fish sandwich
   B. A southwest salad with crispy chicken
   C. A classic grilled chicken sandwich with mayo, lettuce, and tomato

Answer: The winner is the grilled chicken sandwich, at 350 calories and 9 grams of fat. (Try pairing it with a small salad or fruit from home. And ask for the sandwich without mayo and save several more calories.) Meanwhile, don't give me back that Filet-O-Fish, as the commercial goes. It's 380 calories and 18 grams of fat. The vegetables can't redeem the fried chicken in the salad (crispy is restaurant code for high-fat), which will give you 450 calories and 21 grams of fat. (But the same salad with grilled instead of crispy chicken is a good idea—it's 290 calories and 8 grams of fat) [10].

5. **You're at a pizza shop. What are you ordering?**
   A. A pepperoni, ham, and cheese calzone
   B. A plain slice of pizza with a side salad and vinaigrette dressing
   C. A cheesesteak sandwich

Answer: You guessed it. A typical slice of plain cheese pizza is about 272 calories, combined with a side salad and balsamic vinaigrette dressing it's about 422 calories and offers a nice balanced meal. Always choose one slice of pizza and salad, rather than two slices of pizza. Just half of a calzone will give you 641 calories, and a cheese steak will plant 690 calories onto your thighs [11].

6. **You're at a high-end sandwich shop. What are you ordering?**
   A. A bowl of lentil soup
   B. A club sandwich
   C. A grilled salmon salad

Answer: Ten ounces of the lentil soup at Cosi, along with a multigrain flatbread, will give you 472 calories, 6 grams of fat and 18 satisfying grams of fiber. The club sandwich delivers 455 calories, 7 grams of fat, but only 3 grams of fiber. And although it sounds healthy, a grilled salmon salad at Cosi contains 502 calories, 34 grams of fat and a shocking 1,493 milligrams of sodium [12]. As a quick tip, if there is something on the menu that you recognize as being high in fiber (lentils, whole grain, or beans) then that is a good bet, unless it is doused in cheese.

7. **You're at a Mexican restaurant. What are you ordering?**
   A. Chicken fajitas
   B. A taco salad
   C. A classic margarita, which you drink while munching on the free chips and salsa

Answer: If you can skip the rice and beans and eat just one tortilla, the chicken fajitas come in at 430 calories. (That is, if you don't chow down on the chips at the table). A taco salad sounds healthy, but they usually come in crispy, deep-fried flour shells. Even if you get a taco salad with chicken and no dressing at On the Border, you'll still get 1,190 calories and 74 grams of a fat. (Salads can be deceiving. If you add dressing, cheese, and croutons it can cease to be a healthy choice.) And if you think you're saving calories by not ordering a meal and eating chips with a drink, think again. The chips and salsa are 430 calories and 22 grams of fat, and the margarita adds another 153 calories to the total [11, 13].

8. **You're at an Italian restaurant. What are you ordering?**
   A. Eggplant parmesan
   B. Fettuccine alfredo
   C. Pan-seared snapper

Answer: The pan-seared snapper (with sides) at the Macaroni Grill has only 400 calories and fills you up with a healthy protein: fish. You may have guessed that fettuccine alfredo (which has been called a "heart attack on a plate") would blow your eating plan. It clocks in at 770 calories. But the biggest calorie bomb is the eggplant parmesan, at 910 calories [14].

What Works for Me

Sally Koller, home care nurse in Emmaus, PA

My lifestyle became more sedentary in 1996 when my job changed from being a nurse in a hospital setting to caring for patients in their homes. Working in a hospital meant I had a fairly active day walking around to do my job. That stopped once my job required staying in someone's house.

As a result, it's been harder to keep my weight down. I've turned to several commercial weight-loss plans over the years to keep the pounds off, and I've had success with those programs. Recently, I lost fifteen pounds.

(continued)

(*continued*)

When I'm not on a specific weight-loss plan, I've learned a few things to keep my weight in check. One is to give in to cravings in a healthy way. When I want something salty, I'll have a cup of French onion soup or I'll drink V8 juice. When I want something sweet, I'll sink my teeth into a nectarine or I'll enjoy a bowl of strawberries, blueberries, and raspberries.

I've also learned to put half of what I really want to eat on my plate at meal-times. Odds are it's enough to make me feel full and satisfied.

I spend a lot of time taking care of my two grandchildren, but instead of heading to a fast-food restaurant when we want to go out, we take the kids to a sit-down restaurant where we can find healthy options.

I also give myself a splurge day about once a month when I let myself eat whatever I want. I'll go out for a burger, fries, and dessert. Or I'll head to the Olive Garden and eat a salad, ravioli, and a couple of glasses of wine.

The next day, I'm able to go right back to my usual healthy diet. I tend to focus on vegetables, so my typical meals will include tofu, eggs, cheese, yogurt, vegetables, fruit, and whole grains. I love eating a sliced tomato with a little salt, or corn on the cob.

I feel so much better physically and mentally when I'm eating healthy. I think more clearly, I have more energy, and I get through my day without feeling tired or drowsy.

9. **You're at a steakhouse. What are you ordering?**
   A. A 10-ounce New York strip steak with a Caesar salad and mashed potatoes
   B. A 6-ounce sirloin steak with broccoli and tomato salad
   C. An 8-ounce prime rib with a sweet potato and grilled asparagus

Answer: Not surprisingly, the 6-ounce sirloin is the best option. It's on Outback Steakhouse's "Under 500 calories" menu and comes in at 403 calories and 11 grams of fat. The 8-ounce prime rib and sides pack in 895 calories and 31 grams of fat, while the 10-ounce New York strip steak and sides carry 1,183 calories and 80 grams of fat [15]. It's generally best to go for the lean meats and smaller amounts. Then fill up on the veggies and ask your server to hold the sauce or butter.

10. **You're at a bar. What are you ordering?**
    A. A strawberry frozen margarita
    B. A 12-ounce beer
    C. A glass of red wine

Answer: Red wine is probably the best choice because it contains flavanoids and antioxidants that research suggests may protect you from heart disease. However, moderate alcohol consumption in general (up to two drinks a day for men and one drink a day for women) may also be protective. So if you prefer beer, a 12-ounce glass will give you 153 calories (compared to 117 for a glass of wine). The strawberry margarita, on the other hand, has 340 calories [11, 16].

Ready to get started? One more thing. You're getting your environment ready for weight loss. In the next chapter, you'll learn how to set your mind for weight loss. Then you'll be ready.

Dietitian's Diary

Healthy Restaurant Dining

For those of you who think it takes too much time or money to dine in the comfort of your home, I hope we have convinced you of the benefits of preparing your own meals by now. But let's face it, dining out is not just for special occasions anymore. We dine out because we are tired after a long day of work or just don't like to cook. But when you're eating out you don't have to commit nutritional and calorie hara-kiri. Even in a restaurant you can make healthy, satisfying choices.

Here are a few pointers:

Bread

Bread on the table with butter is a common "on-the-house" offering. When dining out, a party of two people can inhale a basket of two to six rolls before they get their main meal and pack on lots of extra calories. Consider the Olive Garden's bread sticks slathered, in garlic butter and packing 150 calories each. So enjoy the bread if you like, but don't feel obligated just because it's free.

Portions

- *Try ordering an appetizer for a meal.*

- *Pick from the children's menu for your meal. No, this is not weird. Children's portions today are what adult portions were years ago.*

- *Choose several healthy options from the sides menu to create a complete meal. I will get a cup of broth-based soup, double side of vegetables, and enjoy a roll from the bread basket. And follow up with a small dessert (see below) if I have a sweet tooth that day.*

- *Then there is the obvious tactic of asking the waiter to bring out a doggie bag with the meal. Turn one restaurant meal into two by eating half at the restaurant and the other half at home tomorrow. Order a 6-ounce filet and eat half of it. Take home the leftover steak and put it on a salad tomorrow. Top with a little vinegar and oil and enjoy again.*

- *If your dining mate agrees, you can always share a meal. Be mindful that some restaurants may charge a plating fee for splitting a meal.*

Go Meatless

- Try a meatless/vegetarian option. Dining out is a great time to try meatless options, especially if you are still learning what types of vegetarian proteins you like and different methods of preparing them.

- Asian restaurants are great places to try tofu.

- Any of the vegetarian options at an Indian restaurant are flavorful and filling.

- Most American diners have vegetarian burgers on their menus now. Ask your server if you can choose a burger on the menu, but substitute a veggie burger in place of the beef.

- Italian food tonight? Give the marinara sauce with eggplant a whirl. The Eggplant Parmesan at Maggiano's has 650 calories, compared to the Chicken Parmesan, which has 1,590 calories [4, 5]. Be sure to watch the cheese for any of these options; too much cheese defeats the purpose of eating less saturated fat from the meat. Use cheese as a condiment, not a meat replacement.

Sides

Substitute, substitute, substitute! Here's a hidden tactic of the restaurant industry: They want you to order fries because it is less expensive for their bottom line and faster to prepare than a baked potato. Remember, you are the customer! The restaurant usually wants to please you in the hope that you return soon. You have every right to substitute a healthier option for your side in place of the fried or less healthy side.

- Try a side salad, double vegetables, or a broth-based soup instead of fries. This substituting practice has become so common that many restaurants have developed different prices for substituting different items.

- Change up the preparation if you can. Order a baked potato, but add vegetables on top (steamed broccoli perhaps) in place of butter. (But remember that a side of vegetables at a restaurant can get high in fat quickly if it is cooked and/or stored in butter in the kitchen. Try asking for no butter on the vegetables and have them steamed or roasted.)

- Go for the brown rice instead of white rice.

- Ask for healthier whole-wheat-flour or corn tortillas instead of regular white-flour tortillas.

- And, of course, get the dressing for the salad on the side.

For a quick solution, watch for the HealthyMeals phone application to be released in January 2012. It will give you a quick view and solution for filling meals on the go, fast food or at a restaurant.

Recipes

PORTOBELLO STEAKS   Serves: 4

4 medium Portobello mushrooms, wiped clean and stem removed
2 tablespoons olive oil, extra virgin
2 tablespoons oregano leaves, dried
2 tablespoons balsamic vinegar
1 tablespoon garlic, minced
4 tablespoons parmesan cheese

Directions:

1. Wipe off mushrooms with wet cloth. Do not run mushrooms under water; this will make them soggy and difficult to cook.
2. Remove stem from mushrooms.
3. Combine oil, garlic, vinegar, and oregano in a bowl.
4. Place steaks on grill or stovetop pan on medium with the top facing down (gills facing you like a bowl).
5. Brush a generous amount of dressing onto each mushroom.
6. Cook through until hot, about 5 minutes.
7. Top with cheese and melt.
8. Serve hot.

   Per serving: 88 calories, 6.9 g fat, 5 g carbohydrate, 0.7 g fiber, 1.4 g fiber.

SATISFACTION SOLUTION CHILI   Serves: 4

1 cup yellow onion, chopped
2 tablespoons garlic, minced
2 tablespoons canola oil
1 package Quorn Grounds
1 15 oz. can red kidney beans, drained and rinsed
2 tablespoons cumin
1 tablespoon chili powder
1 tablespoon cayenne pepper
1 15 oz. can tomatoes, diced
3 tablespoons ketchup

TIP

Quorn is a meatless and soy-free protein source. Check it out at www.quorn.com and find where you can purchase this high-fiber protein source.

Directions:

1. Using a large soup pot, sauté onion and garlic in canola oil.
2. Mix in remaining ingredients and bring to a simmer.
3. On medium heat simmer for about 20 minutes or until heated through.
    Per serving: 353 calories, 10.2 g fat, 43.3 g carbohydrate, 7.9 g fiber, 21.9 g protein.

BLACK BEAN, GREEN SOYBEAN, AND WHEAT BERRY SALAD   Serves: 6

½ cup wheat berries
1 cup frozen soybeans, shelled
1 15 oz. can black beans, drained and rinsed
2 medium Roma tomatoes, chopped
½ cup red onion, diced
3 tablespoons olive oil, extra virgin
2 tablespoons red wine vinegar
Sea salt, to taste
Pepper, fresh ground, to taste

Directions:

1. Cook wheat berries according to package.
2. Rinse frozen soybeans with room temperature water for about one minute to remove frost.
3. Combine all ingredients in a serving bowl and stir. Salt and pepper to taste.
4. Served chilled.

Per serving: 363 calories, 13.6 g fat, 40 g carbohydrate, 3.6 g fiber, 20.2 g protein.

Set Your Mind on Weight Loss

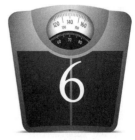

Discover How Powerful Your Own Determination to Succeed Can Be

Of everything you need to lose weight (a food plan, a journal, the right tools), the most important thing is something you can't buy. It comes from you and you alone. You have to believe that you can make changes in your life that will lead to weight loss.

"One of the biggest barriers for people making changes is they don't believe they can do it," says Christy D. Hofsess, PhD.

But the truth is you *can* do it. And most likely, you've already been successful in the past. Most people have been able to exercise at some time in their lives or have been able to follow a food plan for a couple of days or longer.

> *Believing you can change a specific area of your life is called self-efficacy. It's where motivation comes from.*

Ask yourself, what helped you do it in the past? Identifying what works for you and building on successes from the past will help you be successful again, Dr. Hofsess says.

Believing you can change a specific area of your life is called *self-efficacy*. It's where motivation comes from—and it's what will help you put all of the things you're learning about weight loss and how to deal with hunger into practice.

Get Motivated: Believe in Yourself

If you're lacking a little in the self-efficacy department, don't fret. Here's how to build your confidence and get motivated to make this important change in your life.

71

Set Smart, Realistic Goals

One important way to build your confidence is to accomplish something you have set your mind to. That's where goal setting comes into play. But the key is to set achievable goals. We would all like to lose twenty pounds in two weeks, but we know that's just not feasible. Losing weight at a pace that's right for you and your body is best.

To get there, it's essential that you set SMART goals, Dr. Hofsess says. As an acronym, it tells you all the things you need to do to set goals that you'll be able to achieve, and when you do, you'll be building your confidence to lose weight.

- **Specific:** A smart goal is one that's very specific. Instead of saying you want to exercise more, tell yourself you want to start walking.

- **Measurable:** Next, plan how far or how long you're going to walk. If you live near a park with a small lake, you might set a goal of walking one lap around the lake.

- **Attainable:** Be sure this is something you really can do. You wouldn't want to go from being sedentary to running a 5K, for instance.

- **Relevant:** Ask yourself if your goal is going to help you lose weight.

- **Timely:** If you're going to accomplish it, you need to set a time and day when it will fit in your schedule. For example, you might plan to walk for twenty minutes on Monday, Wednesday, and Friday at 6 p.m.

An example of a specific, measurable, attainable, relevant, and timely goal: "I'll walk twenty minutes at Green Lake Tuesday and Thursday after work at 6 p.m. this week."

Other ideas for potential goals (but keep in mind that every goal should be tailored to you):

- Keep a food journal for a single day. Then you'll know you can do it again the next day.

- Take a healthy cooking class or an exercise class.

- Run a mile (or another distance that's a challenge) by starting with walking intervals and building up until you can run the distance.

- Drink more water today.

- Switch out at least one restaurant meal a week with a healthy home-cooked meal.

- Replace your weekly ice cream run with a brisk walk.

- Practice yoga, meditation, or another stress-relief activity.
- Start biking to work.
- Turn off the television at night and go to bed a little earlier.

> When other people believe in you, you're more likely to think you can accomplish anything.

Watch How Others Do It

Watching other people lose weight or make healthy changes in their lives can build your own confidence, Dr. Hofsess says. "That's why groups are effective," she says, such as Overeaters Anonymous or even an online discussion group. When you meet with other people who have the same struggles you do, your experience is normalized. And when you see others skipping Friday happy hour to walk instead, you're more likely to follow suit.

In a recent study in the journal *Obesity*, researchers found that when people who are overweight have friends and family members who are trying to lose weight, it strengthens their intention for weight loss, also [1].

Seek Out a Coach

When other people believe in you, you're more likely to think you can accomplish anything. Tell a friend, parents, a mentor, or a spouse about your goals and ask for support, Dr. Hofsess says.

Harness the Energy Change Brings

Any time you make a change, your body will react. You may feel anxious or physically aroused. "People misinterpret that as a reason not to do something," Dr. Hofsess says. "But it's actually the body's way of giving you an extra boost to do something new."

Do It

Don't overthink it. Just lace up your sneakers and go for a walk or a run. Or drive right by the fast-food joint to make grilled chicken at home. The best way to build your self-efficacy is to just get out there and do it and to have a successful experience. That's what self-efficacy is about.

What Works for Me

Bonnie Matthews, personal trainer, personal chef, motivational weight-loss coach, blogger for the Dr. Oz show (www.doctoroz.com/expert/bonnie-matthews), and regional sales manager and media personality for Nature's Organic Grist in Minneapolis, MN

I lost 130 pounds and kept it off over the last two years by making big changes to the way I eat and live. I gave up the foods that were making me fat, such as pizza and French fries, and started eating lots and lots more vegetables, fruits, lean meats, and whole grains. I also started exercising. At one point I was exercising every single day. Today, I'm a certified personal trainer.

But before I could lose my first pound, I had to really set my mind to it. I started by envisioning what the new me would look like. I thought about the clothes I would wear and how I would carry myself. When I was shopping at the store or walking down the street, I saw women who carried themselves with confidence and grace, and I wanted that for myself.

Jodi Foster's character in the movie *The Brave One* also inspired me. I loved her look and her strong will. She took control of her life, which is something I wanted more than anything.

Day after day of thinking about the person I wanted to become, I started to believe that I was that person. And day after day, I started eating healthier and healthier and moved from being sedentary to active.

The people around me started noticing the pounds slipping away. One day, someone asked me how I did it, and I told her, "You gotta want it more than pizza!"

After two years of a lot of hard work, I weigh half of what I did four years ago. I don't think I could have done it without changing my attitude toward my weight and without visualizing myself at a healthier weight. Today, I'm living the life I dreamed.

For more about Bonnie, go to www.bonniematthews.com

Keep Your Eyes on the Prize

It comes down to this: If you believe you can make healthy changes in your life that will lead to weight loss, you absolutely will. In one Australian study of 564 women between age fifty-one and sixty-six, the researchers found that self-efficacy was one of the most important reasons women gave for exercising and eating healthy. The higher their self-efficacy, the harder the women worked on their goals and the longer they hung in there [2, 3].

Sometimes you need some nudging to stay on track with your goals. In Chapter 1 you read a list of the reasons to lose weight. Now is a good time to make your own personalized list. Think about how much better you'll feel physically once you drop the pounds and the other reasons that are personal to you for wanting to lose weight.

To stay on track, find ways to give yourself encouragement along the way. Melissa Paris writes notes to herself and leaves them in her fridge and in her kitchen cabinets to remind herself of her goals. As a fitness competitor, staying in shape is essential to her career. "In places where I keep food that I tend to want to overeat, I'll post a note that says, 'You're competing June 4,'" she says. Some of her clients also post reminders, such as, "You want healthy skin" or "Keep your energy level up" to remind them why they want to eat healthy [4].

Be sure you use positive, healthy messages, and do your best to ignore negative comments about being overweight. In a study of seventy-three women (who were both overweight and normal weight) researchers broke them up into two groups and showed them a video. One group watched a video that stigmatized weight, and the other saw a video that was neutral about weight. Then the researchers gave the women snacks, took their blood pressure and other measurements, and asked them about their attitude toward people who were overweight [5].

The overweight women who watched the video that stigmatized being overweight ate three times more calories than overweight women who watched the neutral video. They also ate significantly more than women who weren't overweight, regardless of which video the normal weight women watched [5].

So, stay positive and know that you *can* make these healthy changes in your life, and the pounds will just melt away. Hunger will be a friend again instead of your foe.

Sometimes people think their life has to be just right in order to lose weight. They may start eating healthier until work stress interferes and they fall off the wagon. "At some point, you have to make it a regular part of your life," says Amy Wood, PsyD [7]. It's normal to get off track, but you'll gradually learn ways to deal with all of the things that can distract you from your goals without hitting a box of cookies.

Dietitian's Diary

The New MyPlate: A Short History

One simple tool that can help you gear up and stay on track is the new MyPlate from the United States Department of Agriculture (USDA). This is a new take on the USDA's Food Pyramid and much more useful and usable.

The USDA has been our guiding light to nutrition for almost a century. Starting in 1916, the first Food Guide focused on "protective foods" [8]. By the 1940s, it had become the Guide to Good Eating and presented the basic seven food groups as the foundation for nutrient adequacy. But the system proved difficult to understand, so between 1956 and 1970 the basic seven food groups were simplified to the basic four. The new guide was titled Food for Fitness: A Daily Food Guide.

This guide was the first to specify serving sizes of food groups. However, it lacked recommendations on the amounts of fat, sugar, and calories needed for good health. In 1979, the USDA presented the Hassle-Free Daily Food Guide, which included a fifth food group: fats, sweets, and alcohol [7].

To make the guide even simpler, in 1992 the USDA introduced the Food Guide Pyramid with horizontal blocks of different sizes detailing the recommended amounts of each food group. The Food Guide Pyramid was re-invented again in 2005 with vertical sections of different sizes representing the food groups, almost like a pie graph in pyramid form.

Most recently, the USDA has determined that, when it comes to meals, a pyramid is the last shape anyone would actually think about (unless you are playing with your mashed potatoes). This led to the introduction of MyPlate in 2011. The intent of MyPlate, which has changed the pyramid shape to that of a dinner plate, is to help us visually build a healthy plate of food. Finally! Brilliance! It only took ninety-five years, but better late than never.

As a side note, for those vegan-curious, the Physicians Committee for Responsible Medicine uses a similar model as their guide for plant-based dining.

As you'll note in the picture below, there are five basic food groups to have at each meal: whole grains, vegetables, fruits, protein source, and dairy. This book will help you arm yourself with knowledge of the Satisfaction Solution and how to build a healthy plate with your meals and snacks in order to lose and maintain a healthy weight without feeling hungry.

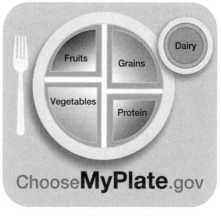

Source: USDA's MyPlate Homepage

Building a Healthy Plate!

Protein on MyPlate: People nine years and older, 5 to 7 ounces a day.

Calcium on MyPlate: Adults need to consume about 300 mg of calcium at each meal or a total of 600 to 800 mg/day.

Fruits and Vegetables on MyPlate: Five to nine servings per day, or roughly two to three servings per meal.

Whole Grains on MyPlate: According to the National Academy of Sciences' Institute of Medicine, we need to consume 22 to 40 grams of fiber a day. This can be from a combination of fruits, vegetables, whole grains, and fiber-fortified foods.

Recipes

CAULIFLOWER TABBOULEH   Serves: 6

1 head cauliflower
2 cups Italian parsley (about one bunch)
2 tablespoons fresh mint leaves
2 green onions
⅓ cup lemon juice, bottled
3 tablespoons olive oil, extra virgin
2 tablespoons soy sauce, low sodium
2 medium Roma tomatoes, chopped
Sea salt and fresh ground pepper, to taste

Directions:

1. Chop all ingredients (except tomatoes) in a food processor with the shredding attachment. Or chop all ingredients by hand if you do not have a food processor.

2. Place in serving bowl and stir in tomatoes to combine.

3. Enjoy cold.

    Per serving: 98 calories, 6.8 g fat, 7 g carbohydrate, 4 g fiber, 2.4 g protein.

GAZPACHO   Serves: 6

¾ cup yellow onion, diced
1 tablespoon garlic, minced
1 green bell pepper, diced

1 yellow bell pepper, diced
1 English cucumber, chopped
2 tablespoons olive oil, extra virgin
1 lime, juiced
zest from 1 medium lime
5 medium tomatoes, chopped
1 cup jicama, diced
1 tablespoon oregano, dried
⅛ teaspoon cumin
1 24 oz. tomato juice, low sodium (one large can)
Pepper, ground, to taste

Directions:

1. Combine all in a bowl.

2. Serve chilled.

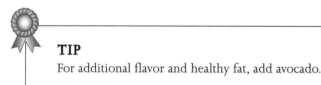

TIP
For additional flavor and healthy fat, add avocado.

Per serving: 121 calories, 5 g fat, 16.4 g carbohydrate, 2.8 g protein.

BEAN SLAW   Serves: 8

1 12 oz. package cabbage coleslaw mix
1 15 oz. can black beans
1 avocado, chopped
¼ cup rice vinegar, seasoned
2 tablespoons olive oil, extra virgin
1 cup cilantro, fresh, chopped
2 tomatoes, chopped
¼ red onion, diced
1 tablespoon cumin
1 lime, juiced

Directions:

1. Combine all ingredients in serving dish.
2. Serve chilled.

Per serving: 174 calories, 7.7 g fat, 19.8 carbohydrate, 2.3 g fiber, 6.2 g protein.

Your Weight-Loss Toolbox

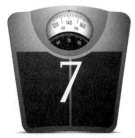

Find Out How To Be Well Equipped for Weight Loss

You wouldn't show up to your first day of a new job without your briefcase, your contact list, or another essential tool that would help you get the job done.

The same goes for weight loss. There is a host of tools out there—from food diaries to the right pots and pans—that can aid you in your weight loss and make the whole process easier and a more satisfying experience.

Getting the right tools means you'll also be ready with everything you need to start digging in and enjoying the meal plans in Part II and the recipes throughout this book. So, let's get started!

Your Number One Tool: A Food Journal

How would you like a tool that can help you *double* the amount of pounds you lose? Something to keep in your back pocket (figuratively and literally) that can help you be as successful as you can possibly be?

It's something as simple as a food journal.

In one of the largest and longest studies about weight loss and weight maintenance, researchers from the Kaiser Permanente Center for Health Research followed almost 1,700 people as they ate a healthy diet and exercised every day. They found that people who kept a food journal every day lost twice as much weight as people who didn't track what they ate [1, 2].

Why is it such a powerful tool for weight loss? For one thing, it may open your eyes to your current eating habits and show you where there's room for improvement. You may notice you're snacking at a certain time of the day or that you're eating bigger portions than what you really need [3].

Knowing all of this will help you schedule your meals and snacks to help you avoid overeating, says Dr. Piotrowski [3].

It also helps give you pause if you keep track of the food in your mouth. You might pick up a handful of peanut butter cups in the middle of the afternoon at work. But if you're determined to write before you eat, you'll get out your food plan and your food journal before popping them in your mouth, says H. Theresa Wright [4].

When you do that, you might say, "I see why I'm hungry. It's time for my afternoon snack," she says. Then it's easier to put down the candy and get the apple and peanut butter you planned for your afternoon snack [4].

As a result, you'll be eating more consciously and mindfully.

You might also find ways to tweak your meals so that they're more satisfying. If you find that you're always overeating at lunch because you're starving by the time you sit down for a meal, you might find that you need to plan heartier and more satisfying breakfasts.

Here's what you should write down in your food diary: the time of day, your hunger rating before eating, the food, the amount of food, where you are, who you're with, the emotions you're feeling at the time, and your hunger rating after eating.

Here's the food diary our dietitian, Crystal Petrello, uses with her clients:

Time of Day/Meal
Hunger Rating Before Meal
Food
Amount
Location
With Whom
Emotions

Hunger Scale Rating

1—Extremely Hungry
2—Hungry
3—Slightly Hungry
4—Almost Satisfied
5—Neutral
6—Satisfied
7—Almost Full
8—Full
9—Very Full
10—Stuffed

The New Food Journal: Not a Single Piece of Paper Needed

If working with a pencil and paper is your preferred way to keep a food journal, go ahead and keep doing that. But technology today offers lots of ways to track what you eat. Send yourself an email or a text of your meals written out, use a food-tracking tool on your computer or smartphone, or create your own spreadsheet or template on your computer to keep track of your food.

Or here's an innovative new way to keep a food journal: Take a picture of your meals and send them to your dietitian.

An online service called MealLogger, designed as a resource for dietitians and their clients, allows you to take a picture of your meals and snacks using your phone or digital camera and send it to your account online. Then your dietitian can review what you're eating and give you feedback about it.

It's quick and simple, and if you *really* want to be accountable for what you eat, photograph it. Seeing an entire day's—or an entire week's or month's—worth of food in full color has a way of sinking in and making an impact on the way you eat, says Nicolas Wuorenheimo, chief technology officer of Wellness Foundry, the company that created MealLogger.

Being able to look at your eating habits at a glance helps you and your dietitian pinpoint habits that are keeping you from losing weight. Maybe you're not eating early enough or setting yourself up for nighttime snacking by going too long during the day without nourishment.

It's also accurate. For a lot of people, writing down their meals is onerous, and they don't include enough information to be accurate. You may write that you ate a small turkey sandwich with cheese, but that doesn't give your dietitian a lot to go on. Inaccuracies can mean your food logs may be off by hundreds of calories.

On the other hand, a picture gives your dietitian a more accurate idea of exactly what you're eating and your portions, especially if you put a set of keys or a pen next to your plate for comparison, Wuorenheimo says. It also holds you accountable to another person and allows your dietitian to give you encouragement on the way you're eating.

And it does one more thing: it makes you slow down your eating long enough to take a picture. In the time it takes to put down the food, get your camera, and click a picture, you may talk yourself out of eating something that wasn't on your food plan.

Tool Number Two: Da-Da-Da-Dum: The Scale— And Other Ways to Monitor Your Progress

If weight has been an issue for you for a while, you probably have a few choice words for your bathroom scale. But the fact is, it's good to have a starting point, says Barbara Mendez.

How often you get on the scale after that first weigh-in is up to you. Some experts recommend weighing yourself once a week at around the same time of day, wearing pretty much the same clothes.

However, getting on the scale sends some people off their eating plan. In Mendez's experience, getting weighed and going shopping are the two key activities that tend to cause people to abandon their weight-loss efforts. That's because some people start to crave sugar or unhealthy food when they're feeling negative—and losing one pound when you expected five can have that effect on you.

> It's probably a good idea to get on the scale regularly, but whether that's weekly, monthly, or quarterly is up to you.

On the other hand, research shows that people who keep track of their weight are more successful. In one study of 348 people conducted by researchers at the Kaiser Permanente Center for Health Research, those who used a website to consistently monitor and log their weight at least once a month for two-and-a-half years were the most successful at maintaining weight loss [5].

It's probably a good idea to get on the scale regularly, but whether that's weekly, monthly, or quarterly is up to you. When you do, make it a good quality digital scale. Digital scales are thought to be more accurate than analog scales [6].

In the meantime, there are plenty of other tools that will help you monitor your progress:

- *A soft fabric tape measure.* Take your bust, chest, waist, and hip measurements once a week and write down (or chart) your progress.

- *A camera.* Take a picture of yourself at the beginning of your weight loss journey and then once a week or once a month to see your progress with your own eyes.

- *Your clothes.* You'll know if you've lost weight based on how your clothes fit and whether or not it's time to shop for a smaller size.

- *A journal.* This time we're not talking about a food journal. This is a place to write down your thoughts and feelings along the way. Every day rate how you feel physically. A couple of months later, it will help to go back and realize exercising every day has improved your knee pain or that you're having fewer tummy problems now that you're eating more fiber.

What Works for Me

Dan Collins, senior director of media relations at Mercy Medical Center in Baltimore, MD

I struggled with my weight throughout adolescence and early adulthood. By the time I graduated from college I weighed 239 pounds. I saw my doctor and told him I wasn't feeling great. He said, "No wonder. You're 239 pounds and your blood pressure is 150/90." He put me on blood-pressure medication and insisted I come to see him once a month to get on a scale and check in.

I was twenty-one at the time. I had a vision of my future and I didn't like it: a five hundred-pound, eternally single guy living in his parents' basement. That was not going to be me.

Up to that point, I was able to stay in retreat of life. My home and family served as a shield between reality and myself. Once I finished college, I knew I had to leave the nest, lest I become an obese geek-basement-troll. I was going to have to deal with people, and let's face it, we are judged by our appearance in American society.

At that moment, I was committed. I went back to my doctor for the weigh-ins and over the next two years I got my weight down to 183, which he thought was a good weight for me at five-feet-eleven-inches.

That was a quarter of a century ago. Although I'm in the low 190s now, I go to the gym at least three times a week and fence with the Chesapeake Fencing Club.

My advice for losing weight is pretty simple: you have to really want it. No, that's not right. You need to really, really—I mean *really*—want to lose weight. If you're not fully committed, you won't succeed. Believe me, nobody can make you lose weight.

Today, I look back, and I know vanity proved helpful. I like looking good, and I like that losing weight made me attractive to the opposite sex. (Sorry, if you're obese and you're not a Bill Gates or a highly successful rap artist, chances are you're going to the prom alone.)

I learned that I had to irrevocably change how I ate. It wasn't a diet, because that would mean that once I was off the diet I'd gain the weight back. I still eat pretty much whatever I want, but instead of having eight scoops of ice cream, I have one.

The hardest part about losing weight is the beginning. Creating new eating and exercise habits is hard because you're trying to break old habits and addictions. But if you can tough out those early weeks, you'll be rewarded. It does get easier as you go along, and once you've settled into a new groove of healthy eating and exercise, you'll find that it becomes a habit you won't want to quit.

Tool Number Three: A Stocked Pantry

Here's what you're going to need to have on hand to make the healthy recipes in this book.

- Bottled sundried tomatoes packed with oil
- Jarred roasted red peppers
- Jarred marinated artichoke hearts
- Healthy oils: olive and canola
- Vinegars: white balsamic, seasoned rice, apple cider, red wine
- Canned beans: black beans, kidney beans, chick peas, navy beans, or cannellini beans
- Sea salt
- Pepper
- Spices
- Dried herbs
- Several Mrs. Dash seasoning varieties
- Honey and/or agave syrup
- Plain nuts of all types
- Nut butters (natural is more preferable, nothing with partially hydrogenated oils/trans fats)
- Seeds
- Raisins and other dried fruits
- Brown rice
- Oatmeal
- Whole-wheat pasta
- Whole-wheat flour
- Variety of fresh fruits and vegetables for snacking
- Extracts, including brandy extract
- Flaxseed meal
- Liquid smoke
- TVP, textured vegetable protein

SATISFACTION SOLUTION TIP
Vinegar, herbs, and spices add lots of flavor to meat, vegetables, and salads without packing on calories and fat.

SATISFACTION SOLUTION TIP
Sea salt is unrefined and is made by evaporating seawater, which makes it more flavorful than table salt. Because it has more flavor, you'll be able to get away with using less. However, it's coarser than table salt, so you may want to grind it [7]. (And don't worry about not getting enough iodine. It's also found in milk, egg yolks, and saltwater fish.)

Satisfaction Solution Tools

Cooking at home means you have complete control over every ingredient in your meal. These tools will make home-prepared meals easier.

Must-Haves

These items are the basic tools for healthy cooking. You may have most already. If you don't, it's a good idea to try stocking your kitchen with these tools so you're equipped and ready to make the recipes throughout the book and meals in Part 2. Don't use a lack of this equipment as an excuse for not reaching your goal. You can gather implements over time and, in the meantime, you can borrow them from neighbors. Also, check out yard sales for inexpensive implements.

- Good knife for chopping vegetables
- Serrated knife for slicing bread
- Kitchen shears for cutting herbs, scallions, and meat
- Measuring spoons and cups

- Zester
- Nonstick pans
- Stock pot for making soup
- Cookie sheets for roasting vegetables
- A roasting pan
- Inexpensive plastic cutting boards (one for meat, one for fish, one for vegetables)
- Mixing bowls of various sizes
- Colander
- Meat thermometer
- Kitchen food scale
- A folder, binder, or box to store healthy recipes
- A salt mill or grinder

Dream List

These tools make life a little easier, but they're not necessities if they don't fit in your budget.

- Salad spinner for drying lettuce, veggies, and berries
- Blender for making smoothies or pureeing creamy soups
- Full-size food processor or mini chopper
- Full-size mixer or hand-held electric beaters
- Outdoor grill or stovetop grill pan

On-the-Go Satisfaction Solutions

You already know that it's just as important to be prepared when you leave the house. These items will help.

- A reusable lunch bag for work
- Plastic baggies and reusable containers that can go in the freezer
- A small cooler to keep wraps, sandwiches, veggies, and fruit fresh during road trips

📖 Dietitian's Diary

Pantry Raid Recipes

Let's say you have a good amount of food in the house, but it is mostly leftover ingredients from previous recipes, none of which you have all of the ingredients for. You have also already gotten into your comfy clothes and don't feel like going out to the grocery store. What would you do? Would you call the Pizza Man? At my house we stage our own culinary battle, "Pantry Wars." My husband and I compete to see who can make the most delicious meal with items from the pantry. The stipulations change from time to time, but the main rules are always the same:

- The meal must be considered a "complete" meal.
- The whole meal must be made from ingredients already at the house.
- No re-creating a meal from the previous five days.
- Overall taste is the main factor for victory, but using the most items gets bonus points.
- Bottom line: We save money and use all this food!

Here are the steps I go through to dominate my competition:

1. Think of the MyPlate and build a meal around the picture of a balanced meal: whole grains, vegetables, and lean meat/vegetarian protein option.

2. Find one item from each of these groups. Always pair with a dairy/calcium source and fruit for dessert.

3. Pick a general flavor for the meal. This usually is the overall theme of the meal. Remember, you can use pasta to make an Asian dish just as simply as you can an Italian dish.

4. Cook-up:
   a. If you are looking to save time or want less to clean, choose a one-pot meal. This can be a hearty stew, risotto, or stir-fry.
   b. If the pantry war is pre-planned: crock pot. All you need is a little liquid and seasoning on your meat and it will be to-temperature by the time you get home from work. Or, eliminate having to soak your dried beans. Wash and sift the beans (as usual), cover about two inches above beans with liquid of choice, and add seasoning. You can add vegetables when you get home and BOOM, a delicious stew! Serve over wheat berries for a satisfying meal.
   c. Try cooking each item at the same time, but in different areas of the kitchen. Cook the thawed meat on the stove, steam the vegetables in the microwave, and put the couscous in the rice steamer. Dinner in less than thirty minutes. Just add herbs.
   d. Semi-homemade pizza: Have a cheese pizza handy (or wheat dough if you have decided by now to eat less cheese) and add as many vegetables as you desire. Cook pizza with

vegetables atop (this may need more time to cook). This way you cook the vegetables and pizza at the same time. No tomato sauce in the pantry? Try barbecue or teriyaki sauce.

Here are a few more of my favorite pantry-raid creations:

- Leftover pork, frozen broccoli, and corn (rinsed to quickly thaw) stir-fried with garlic and Asian sweet chili sauce. Serve over whole-wheat pasta.

- Cheese pizza with zucchini, left over barbeque chicken, and canned pineapple, with a side salad and piece of fruit.

- A bag of pinto beans covered in vegetable broth cooked in the crock pot on high for six hours. Make tacos with beans, tomatoes, salsa, avocado, and some cheese. Add a side salad, of course! Take the same pinto beans and puree in a blender or food processor. Use that for a dip with vegetables the next day.

- Microwave baked potatoes and load with cooked broccoli and little shredded cheese. Add pan-cooked chicken with Tomato Basil Garlic Mrs. Dash. Add more broccoli on the side to make sure you get enough greens!

Live

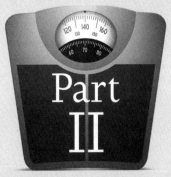

Part
II

Introducing the Satisfaction Solution

Americans don't have a good track record for the way we eat to lose weight. Deprivation has been the trend, especially among fad diets like the cabbage soup diet, the grapefruit diet, or the baby food diet. Then there are fad diets that promote deprivation disguised as indulgence, like the Twinkies diet or the chocolate diet [1, 2].

Any weight loss that results from a fad diet happens because of calorie restriction, but who can eat nothing but cabbage or grapefruit, or even chocolate, for longer than a couple of days? If you do stay on a fad diet for more than a few weeks, you're setting yourself up for nutritional deficiencies [3].

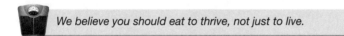

We believe you should eat to thrive, not just to live.

Why do them? Maybe because too many people are convinced they can't lose weight without feeling hungry, so if a fad diet does the trick, why not snack on Twinkies all day?

We're here to tell you: It's not true. You *can* lose weight without being hungry, and you most definitely don't have to—and shouldn't—eat one food all day long.

When you do it the right way you not only satisfy your hunger but you also get all the nutrition you need. Eating to feel full means tapping into what we call the Satisfaction Solution. We believe you should eat to thrive, not just to live.

The Satisfaction Solution is the element about a meal or snack that helps you feel full and lose weight. Tapping into the Satisfaction Solution means eating breakfast; planning a snack or meal every two to four hours; balancing your meals with a variety of foods; getting enough sleep; lowering your stress level; and getting enough protein, fat, fiber, and water. (Each of these Satisfaction Solutions is covered in Chapters 8 through 15.) This may sound like a full-time endeavor, but we're here to help you with an easy-to-follow, step-by-step plan for making these important changes in your life.

The meal plans and the recipes throughout the book have one or more Satisfaction Solutions built in. The meals are filled with fiber and are balanced for good health.

But as you follow the meal plans and make the recipes, there's more you can do to put an end to hunger pangs, from sipping water between meals to going to bed early. And when you're planning your own meals or eating out, knowing how to build in Satisfaction Solutions like fiber and the right amount of fat will help you be a weight-loss success. Think of the recipes and meal plans we offer as snapshots of your new life plan.

Meal Plans

We've created sample meal plans ranging from a 1,600-calorie-per-day plan to a sample menu for 2,500 calories. To determine which meal plan to follow, perform this simple calculation: Multiply your current weight in pounds by ten or twelve. For example, a 180-pound person should consume about 1,800–2,160 calories. Start with the lower amount on the range and if you are still hungry then add some healthy calories.

The total calorie-count for each plan is within 25 calories of the goal. Fat makes up 25 to 30 percent of total daily calories, carbohydrates account for 55 percent, with protein making 15 percent of total calories. Each plan provides at least 25 grams of fiber a day. (Protein, carbs, fat, and fiber are measured in grams.)

Obviously, we want you to view the plans as merely suggestions—possible ways to get started on your new, healthy lifestyle. We hope you'll use them as guides, then make them your own by adding your own favorite recipes. (You'll find page numbers next to each But I'm Hungry! recipe.) Note: Any plan would work for any day of the week. We organized them under specific days of the week simply for the sake of organization.

The plans start on the next page, so you're off …

1,600-Calorie Meal Plans: Sunday

		Protein	Carbs	Fat	Fiber	Calories
Breakfast	Breakfast Smoothie (Page 247)	10.20	34.4	5.59	3.8	229
	½ slice whole-grain toast	1.75	5.65	0.55	1	34.5
	½ tablespoon peanut butter	2.00	1.75	4	0.25	47.75
Lunch	Shrimp Taco (Page 15)	11.75	19.3	1.75	1.5	140.5
	2 tablespoons avocado	0.00	0	5	3	45

		Protein	Carbs	Fat	Fiber	Calories
	2 cups salad	4.00	10	0	8	50
	1 tablespoon vinegar	0.00	0	0	0	25
	Cilantro Soup (Page 256)	1.00	35.1	0.59	1.44	150
Dinner	Asian Flank Steak (Page 245)	12.20	5.9	13	0.15	190
	Cucumber Salad (Page 244)	1.25	11	3.75	0.4	83
	One sandwich thin-two halves, whole wheat	5.00	21	1	6	100
	1 serving fruit	0.00	15	0	3	60
Snack	Bean Slaw (Page 78)	6.23	19.8	7.7	2.28	174
	1 cup strawberries	0.00	15	0	0	60
Quick Snack	Corn and Avocado Dip (Page 255)	3.90	16.3	8.05	2	152
	2 cups raw vegetables	4.00	10	0	8	50
	Totals	63.28	220.20	50.98	40.82	1,590.75

1,600-Calorie Meal Plans: Monday

		Protein	Carbs	Fat	Fiber	Calories
Breakfast	Baked Oatmeal Casserole (Page 246)	7.80	50.4	8.1	2.26	307
Lunch	Brie and Pear sandwich (Page 14)	21.90	35	10.9	7.1	327

(Continued)

		Protein	Carbs	Fat	Fiber	Calories
	Cauliflower Tabbouleh (Page 77)	2.30	6.97	6.79	0.95	98
	Greek yogurt, plain, ½ cup	7.50	3	0	0	40
	1 tablespoon honey	0.00	17	0	0	60
Dinner	Smoky Corn Risotto (Page 189)	4.80	59.2	10	3.79	348
	1 cup cooked vegetables	4.00	10	0	8	50
Snack	Hearts of Palm Salad (Page 250)	3.90	9.1	14.5	2.39	183
	1 serving fruit	0.00	15	0	2	60
Quick Snack	Tofu Dip, 2 servings (Page 256)	6.88	4.48	2.03	0.06	82
	2 cups raw vegetables	4.00	10	0	8	50
	Totals	63.08	220.15	52.33	34.55	1,605.00

1,600-Calorie Meal Plans: Tuesday

		Protein	Carbs	Fat	Fiber	Calories
Breakfast	Figgy Quinoa Pudding (Page 44)	6.40	32.9	2.6	2.15	181

		Protein	Carbs	Fat	Fiber	Calories
	⅓ – ½ cup 100% fruit juice	0.00	15	0	0	60
Lunch	Gazpacho (Page 77)	2.76	16.4	4.95	1.8	121
	Sweet Mexican Salad (Page 256)	10.00	42.8	0.92	3.3	220
	1 tablespoon avocado	0.00	0	5	3	45
Dinner	Baked Breaded Salmon (Page 246)	23.50	17.7	8.2	0.1	239
	Walnut Pesto (Page 171)	3.00	4.1	16.1	1.59	173
	1 cup cooked vegetables	4.00	10	0	8	50
	⅓ cup cooked brown rice	3.00	15	1		80
	½ serving fruit	0.00	7.5	0	1.5	30
Snack	Black Bean Dip (Page 201)	4.90	14.7	0.31	1.1	81
	2 cups raw vegetables	4.00	10	0	8	50

(Continued)

		Protein	Carbs	Fat	Fiber	Calories
Quick Snack	1 ounce almonds	6.00	0	14	3.3	164
	4 tablespoons dried fruit	0.00	30	0		120
	Totals	67.56	216.10	53.08	33.84	1,614.00

1,600-Calorie Meal Plans: Wednesday

		Protein	Carbs	Fat	Fiber	Calories
Breakfast	Fruited Oatmeal (Page 148)	8.30	32.2	13.3	2.48	282
	1 serving fruit	0.00	15	0	3	60
Lunch	Black Bean and Wheat Berry Salad (Page 70)	20.00	40	13.5	3.6	363
	2 cups mixed greens	4.00	10	0	4	50
	1 serving fruit	0.00	15	0	3	60
Dinner	Cajun Jambalaya (Page 42)	18.30	60.8	8.18	1.9	390
	½ cup cooked vegetables	2.00	5	0	3	25
Snack	Tortilla Salad (Page 257)	5.90	23.9	3.6	1.96	152
Quick Snack	2 tablespoons dried fruit	0.00	15	0	3	60

	Protein	Carbs	Fat	Fiber	Calories
1 ounce almonds	6.00	0	14	3.3	164
Totals	64.50	216.90	52.58	29.24	1,606.00

1,600-Calorie Meal Plans: Thursday

		Protein	Carbs	Fat	Fiber	Calories
Breakfast	Fruited Granola (Page 150)	9.70	54.9	5.1	5	305
Lunch	Satisfaction Solution Wrap (Page 254)	18.10	26.8	20.9	8.7	368
	Watermelon Salad (Page 258)	0.78	13.58	0.5	0.4	62
	Greek yogurt, plain, ½ cup	7.50	3	0	0	40
	½ – ¾ cup berries	0.00	15	0	3	60
Dinner	Fajita Pasta (Page 159)	15.20	55.6	8.78	2.66	363
	2 cups raw vegetable salad	4.00	10	0	3	50
	1 tablespoon vinegar	0.00	0	0	0	29
	½ tablespoon oil	0.00	0	2.25	0	20
Snack	Black-Eyed Pea Salad (Page 255)	6.10	21.3	2.25	1.4	130

(Continued)

		Protein	Carbs	Fat	Fiber	Calories
Quick Snack	1 serving fruit	0.00	15	0	2	60
	1 tablespoon peanut butter	4.00	3.5	8	0.5	95.5
	Totals	65.38	218.68	47.78	26.66	1,582.50

1,600-Calorie Meal Plans: Friday

		Protein	Carbs	Fat	Fiber	Calories
Breakfast	Breakfast Frittata (Page 234)	15.20	17.65	13.45	1	253
	1 serving fruit	0.00	15	0	3	60
	⅓–½ cup 100% fruit juice	0.00	15	0	0	60
Lunch	Tangy Peach and Whole Grain Salad (Page 29)	7.97	38	10.9	2	282
	3 cups raw leafy greens	6.00	15	0	6	75
	1 serving fruit	0.00	15	0	3	60
Dinner	Parsnips (and Pork Loin) (Page 252)	9.79	62	4.9	4.49	332
	2 ounces pork loin	14.80	0	2	0	81
Snack	2 cups raw celery	4	10	0	8	50

		Protein	Carbs	Fat	Fiber	Calories
	2 tablespoons peanut butter	8.00	7	16	1	191
Quick Snack	Greek Salad (Page 250)	3.50	32	4	1	179
	Totals	69.26	226.65	51.25	29.49	1,623.00

1,600-Calorie Meal Plans: Saturday

		Protein	Carbs	Fat	Fiber	Calories
Breakfast	Heirloom Benedict (Page 159)	13.20	30.5	14.1	7.8	302
	1 serving fruit	0.00	15	0	3	60
Lunch	Satisfaction Solution Salad (Page 30)	11.45	32.5	9.6	4.1	262
	White Beans and Pesto (Page 258)	4.50	12	1	0.6	77
	1 serving fruit	0.00	15	0	3	60
	Black olives, 4	0.20	1.39	2.1	0.7	24
Dinner	Baked Crispy Chicken (Page 190)	20.75	25.6	9.3	0.09	270
	Pumpkin Pancakes (Page 235)	5.98	24.1	1.7	4.35	136

(Continued)

		Protein	Carbs	Fat	Fiber	Calories
	Light maple syrup, 2 tablespoons	0.00	13.5	0	0.5	52
Snack	Tofu Dip, 1 serving (Page 256)	3.44	2.24	1	0.03	41
	1 cup raw vegetables	2.00	5	0	4	25
	½ cup applesauce	0.00	7	0		30
Quick Snack	1 ounce almonds	6.00	0	14	3.3	164
	4 tablespoons dried fruit	0.00	30	0		120
	Totals	67.52	213.83	52.78	31.47	1,623.00

1,800-Calorie Meal Plans: Sunday

		Protein	Carbs	Fat	Fiber	Calories
Breakfast	Breakfast Smoothie (Page 247)	10.20	34.4	5.59	3.8	229
	1 slice whole grain toast	3.50	11.3	1.1	1.9	69
	1 tablespoon peanut butter	4.00	3.5	8	0.5	95.5
	1 serving fruit	0.00	15	0	3	60
Lunch	Shrimp Taco (Page 15)	11.75	19.3	1.75	1.5	140.5
	2 tablespoons avocado	0.00	0	5	3	45
	3 cups salad	6.00	15	0	12	75
	1 tablespoon vinegar	0.00	0	0	0	25

		Protein	Carbs	Fat	Fiber	Calories
	Cilantro Soup (Page 256)	1.00	35.1	0.59	1.44	150
Dinner	Asian Flank Steak (Page 245)	12.20	5.9	13	0.15	190
	Cucumber Salad (Page 244)	1.25	11	3.75	0.4	83
	One sandwich thin-two halves, whole wheat	5.00	21	1	6	100
	1 serving fruit	0.00	15	0	3	60
Snack	Bean Slaw (Page 78)	6.23	19.8	7.7	2.28	174
	1 cup nonfat milk	8.00	12	1	0	100
Quick Snack	Corn and Avocado Dip (Page 255)	3.90	16.3	8.05	2	152
	2 cups raw vegetables	4.00	10	0	8	50
	Totals	77.03	244.60	56.53	48.97	1,798.00

1,800-Calorie Meal Plans: Monday

		Protein	Carbs	Fat	Fiber	Calories
Breakfast	Baked Oatmeal Casserole (Page 246)	7.80	50.4	8.1	2.26	307
	1 cup nonfat milk	8.00	12	1	0	100

(Continued)

		Protein	Carbs	Fat	Fiber	Calories
Lunch	Brie and Pear Sandwich (Page 14)	21.90	35	10.9	7.1	327
	Cauliflower Tabbouleh (Page 77)	2.30	6.97	6.79	0.95	98
	Greek yogurt, plain, 1 cup	15.00	6	0	0	80
	1 tablespoon honey	0.00	17	0	0	60
Dinner	Smoky Sweet Corn Risotto (Page 189)	4.80	59.2	10	3.79	348
	1 cup cooked vegetables	4.00	10	0	8	50
Snack	Hearts of Palm Salad (Page 250)	3.90	9.1	14.5	2.39	183
	1 serving fruit	0.00	15	0	2	60
Quick Snack	Tofu Dip, 2 servings (Page 256)	6.88	4.48	2.03	0.06	82
	2 cups raw vegetables	4.00	10	0	8	50
	½ cup nonfat milk	4.00	6	0.5	0	50
	Totals	82.58	241.15	53.83	34.55	1,795.00

1,800-Calorie Meal Plans: Tuesday

		Protein	Carbs	Fat	Fiber	Calories
Breakfast	Figgy Quinoa Pudding (Page 44)	6.40	32.9	2.6	2.15	181

		Protein	Carbs	Fat	Fiber	Calories
	1 serving fruit	0.00	15	0	0	60
	1 cup nonfat milk	8.00	12	1	0	100
Lunch	Gazpacho (Page 77)	2.76	16.4	4.95	1.8	121
	Sweet Mexican Salad (Page 256)	10.00	42.8	0.92	3.3	220
	4 tablespoons avocado	0.00	0	10	6	90
Dinner	Baked Breaded Salmon (Page 246)	23.50	17.7	8.2	0.1	239
	Walnut Pesto (Page 171)	3.00	4.1	16.1	1.59	173
	1 cup cooked vegetables	4.00	10	0	8	50
	⅓ cup cooked brown rice	3.00	15	1		80
	½ serving fruit	0.00	7.5	0	1.5	30
Snack	Black Bean Dip (Page 201)	4.90	14.7	0.31	1.1	81
	3 cups raw vegetables	6.00	15	0	12	75
	1 serving fruit	0.00	15	0	3	60

(Continued)

		Protein	Carbs	Fat	Fiber	Calories
Quick Snack	1 ounce peanuts	6.70	6.1	14	3.25	166
	2 tablespoons dried fruit	0.00	15	0	3	60
	Totals	78.26	239.20	59.08	46.79	1,786.00

1,800-Calorie Meal Plans: Wednesday

		Protein	Carbs	Fat	Fiber	Calories
Breakfast	Fruited Oatmeal (Page 148)	8.30	32.2	13.3	2.48	282
	1 serving fruit	0.00	15	0	3	60
	1 cup nonfat milk	8.00	12	1	0	100
Lunch	Black Bean and Wheat Berry Salad (Page 70)	20.00	40	13.5	3.6	363
	2 cups mixed greens	4.00	10	0	4	50
	1 serving fruit	0.00	15	0	3	60
Dinner	Cajun Jambalaya (Page 42)	18.30	60.8	8.18	1.9	390
	½ cup cooked vegetables	2.00	5	0	3	25
Snack	Tortilla Salad (Page 257)	5.90	23.9	3.6	1.96	152

		Protein	Carbs	Fat	Fiber	Calories
	Greek yogurt, plain, ½ cup	7.50	3	0	0	40
Quick Snack	¼ cup dried fruit	0.00	30	0	6	120
	1 ounce almonds	6.00	0	14	3.3	164
	Totals	80.00	246.90	53.58	32.24	1,806.00

1,800-Calorie Meal Plans: Thursday

		Protein	Carbs	Fat	Fiber	Calories
Breakfast	Fruited Granola (Page 150)	9.70	54.9	5.1	5	305
Lunch	Satisfaction Solution Wrap (Page 254)	18.10	26.8	20.9	8.7	368
	Watermelon Salad (Page 258)	0.78	13.58	0.5	0.4	62
	Greek Yogurt, plain, 1 cup	15.00	6	0	0	80
	½–¾ cup berries	0.00	15	0	3	60
Dinner	Fajita Pasta (Page 159)	15.20	55.6	8.78	2.66	363
	2 cups raw vegetable salad	4.00	10	0	3	50

(Continued)

		Protein	Carbs	Fat	Fiber	Calories
	½ tablespoon vinegar	0.00	0	0	0	14.5
	½ tablespoon oil	0.00	0	2.25	0	20
Snack	Black-Eyed Pea Salad (Page 255)	6.10	21.3	2.25	1.4	130
	1 serving fruit	0.00	15	0	2	60
	1 tablespoon peanut butter	4.00	3.5	8	0.5	95.5
Quick Snack	3 cups raw vegetables	6.00	15	0	12	75
	3 tablespoons light salad dressing	0.00	10.5	9	0	120
	Totals	78.88	247.18	56.78	38.66	1,803.00

1,800-Calorie Meal Plans: Friday

		Protein	Carbs	Fat	Fiber	Calories
Breakfast	Breakfast Frittata (Page 234)	15.20	17.65	13.45	1	253
	1 tablespoon honey	0.00	17	0	0	60
	Greek yogurt, plain, ½ cup	7.00	3	0	0	40
	⅓ – ½ cup fruit juice	0.00	15	0	0	60
Lunch	Tangy Peach and Whole Grain Salad (Page 29)	7.97	38	10.9	2	282

		Protein	Carbs	Fat	Fiber	Calories
	3 cups raw leafy greens	6.00	15	0	6	75
	1 serving fruit	0.00	15	0	3	60
Dinner	Parsnips and Pork Loin (Page 252)	9.79	62	4.9	4.49	332
	2 ounces pork loin	14.80	0	2	0	81
Snack	Greek Salad (Page 250)	3.50	32	4	1	179
	1 ounce almonds	6.00	0	14	3.3	164
Quick Snack	2 cups raw celery	4	10	0	8	50
	1 tablespoon peanut butter	4.00	3.5	8	0.5	95.5
	2 tablespoons dried fruit	0.00	15	0	3	60
	Totals	78.26	243.15	57.25	32.29	1,791.50

1,800-Calorie Meal Plans: Saturday

		Protein	Carbs	Fat	Fiber	Calories
Breakfast	Heirloom Benedict (Page 159)	13.20	30.5	14.1	7.8	302
	1 serving fruit	0.00	15	0	3	60

(Continued)

		Protein	Carbs	Fat	Fiber	Calories
	½ cup nonfat milk	4.00	6	0.5	0	50
Lunch	Satisfaction Solution Salad (Page 30)	11.45	32.5	9.6	4.1	262
	White Beans and Pesto (Page 258)	4.50	12	1	0.6	77
	1 serving fruit	0.00	15	0	3	60
	Black olives, 8	0.40	2.79	4.3	1.4	48
Dinner	Baked Crispy Chicken (Page 190)	20.75	25.6	9.3	0.09	270
	Pumpkin Pancakes (Page 235)	5.98	24.1	1.7	4.35	136
	Light maple syrup, 2 tablespoons	0.00	13.5	0	0.5	52
Snack	Tofu Dip, 2 servings (Page 256)	6.88	4.48	2	0.06	82
	3 cups raw vegetables	6.00	15	0	10	75
	1 serving fruit	0.00	15	0	3	60
Quick Snack	¼ cup dried fruit	0.00	30	0	6	120
	1 ounce almonds	6.00	0	14	3.3	164
	Totals	79.16	241.47	56.48	47.20	1,818.00

2,000-Calorie Meal Plans: Sunday

		Protein	Carbs	Fat	Fiber	Calories
Breakfast	Breakfast Smoothie	10.20	34.4	5.59	3.8	229
	1 slice whole grain toast	3.50	11.3	1.1	1.9	69
	1 tablespoon peanut butter	4.00	3.5	8	0.5	95.5
	1 serving fruit	0.00	15	0	3	60
Lunch	Shrimp Tacos, 2 (Page 15)	23.50	38.6	3.5	3	281
	4 tablespoons avocado	0.00	0	10	6	90
	1.5 cups salad	3.00	7.5	0	4.5	39.5
	1 tablespoon vinegar	0.00	0	0	0	25
	Cilantro Soup (Page 256)	1.00	35.1	0.59	1.44	150
Dinner	Asian Flank Steak (Page 245)	12.20	5.9	13	0.15	190
	Cucumber Salad (Page 244)	1.75	11	3.75	0.4	83
	One sandwich thin-two halves, whole wheat	5.00	21	1	6	100
	1 serving fruit	0.00	15	0	3	60
	Greek yogurt, plain, ½ cup	7.50	3	0	0	40

(Continued)

		Protein	Carbs	Fat	Fiber	Calories
	1 tablespoon honey	0.00	17	0	0	60
Snack	Bean Slaw (Page 78)	6.23	19.8	7.7	2.28	174
	½ cup nonfat milk	4.00	6	2	0	50
Quick Snack	Corn and Avocado Dip (Page 255)	3.90	16.3	8.05	2	152
	2 cups raw vegetables	4.00	10	0	8	50
	Totals	89.78	270.40	64.28	45.97	1,998.00

2,000-Calorie Meal Plans: Monday

		Protein	Carbs	Fat	Fiber	Calories
Breakfast	Baked Oatmeal Casserole (Page 246)	7.80	50.4	8.1	2.26	307
	1 cup nonfat milk	8.00	12	1	0	100
Lunch	Brie and Pear sandwich (Page 14)	21.90	35	10.9	7.1	327
	Cauliflower Tabbouleh (Page 77)	2.30	6.97	6.79	0.95	98
	Greek yogurt, plain, 1 cup	15.00	6	0	0	80
	1 tablespoon honey	0.00	17	0	0	60
	1 serving fruit	0.00	15	0	3	60

		Protein	Carbs	Fat	Fiber	Calories
Dinner	Smoky Sweet Corn Risotto (Page 189)	4.80	59.2	10	3.79	348
	2 cups cooked vegetables	8.00	20	0	16	100
	1 tablespoon butter/ margarine	0.00	0	11.5	0	102
Snack	Hearts of Palm Salad (Page 250)	3.90	9.1	14.5	2.39	183
	1 serving fruit	0.00	15	0	2	60
Quick Snack	Tofu Dip, 2 servings (Page 256)	6.88	4.48	2.03	0.06	82
	2 cups raw vegetables	4.00	10	0	8	50
	½ cup nonfat milk	4.00	6	0.5	0	50
	Totals	86.58	266.15	65.33	45.55	2,007.00

2,000-Calorie Meal Plans: Tuesday

		Protein	Carbs	Fat	Fiber	Calories
Breakfast	Figgy Quinoa Pudding (Page 44)	6.40	32.9	2.6	2.15	181
	1 serving fruit	0.00	15	0	0	60
	1 cup nonfat milk	8.00	12	1	0	100

(Continued)

		Protein	Carbs	Fat	Fiber	Calories
Lunch	Gazpacho, 2 servings (Page 77)	5.52	32.8	9.9	3.6	242
	Sweet Mexican Salad (Page 256)	10.00	42.8	0.92	3.3	220
	4 tablespoons avocado	0.00	0	10	6	90
Dinner	Baked Breaded Salmon (Page 246)	23.50	17.7	8.2	0.1	239
	Walnut Pesto (Page 171)	3.00	4.1	16.1	1.59	173
	2 cups cooked vegetables	8.00	20	0	16	100
	⅓ cup cooked brown rice	3.00	15	1		80
	1 serving fruit	0.00	15	0	3	60
Snack	Black Bean Dip (Page 201)	4.90	14.7	0.31	1.1	81
	3 cups raw vegetables	6.00	15	0	12	75
	1 serving fruit	0.00	15	0	3	60
Quick Snack	1 ounce peanuts	6.70	6.1	14	3.25	166
	2 tablespoon dried fruit	0.00	15	0	3	60
	Totals	85.02	273.10	64.03	58.09	1,987.00

2,000-Calorie Meal Plans: Wednesday

		Protein	Carbs	Fat	Fiber	Calories
Breakfast	Fruited Oatmeal (Page 148)	8.30	32.2	13.3	2.48	282
	1 serving fruit	0.00	15	0	3	60
	½ cup nonfat milk	4.00	6	0.5	0	50
Lunch	Black Bean and Wheat Berry Salad (Page 70)	20.00	40	13.5	3.6	363
	3 cups mixed greens	6.00	15	0	6	75
	1 serving fruit	0.00	15	0	3	60
	1 tablespoon peanut butter	4.00	3.5	8	0.5	95.5
Dinner	Cajun Jambalaya (Page 42)	18.30	60.8	8.18	1.9	390
	1 ½ cups cooked vegetables	6.00	15	0	12	75
	½ cup nonfat milk	4.00	6	2	0	50
Snack	Tortilla Salad (Page 257)	5.90	23.9	3.6	1.96	152
	Greek yogurt, plain, ½ cup	7.50	3	0	0	40
Quick Snack	¼ cup dried fruit	0.00	30	0	6	120

(Continued)

	Protein	Carbs	Fat	Fiber	Calories
1 ounce almonds	6.00	0	14	3.3	164
Totals	90.00	265.40	63.08	43.74	1,976.50

2,000-Calorie Meal Plans: Thursday

		Protein	Carbs	Fat	Fiber	Calories
Breakfast	Fruited Granola (Page 150)	9.70	54.9	5.1	5	305
	½ serving fruit	0.00	7.5	0	1.5	30
Lunch	Satisfaction Solution Wrap (Page 254)	18.10	26.8	20.9	8.7	368
	Watermelon Salad, 2 servings (Page 258)	1.56	27.6	1	0.8	124
	Greek yogurt, plain, 1cup	15.00	6	0	0	80
	1 tablespoon honey	0.00	17	0	0	60
Dinner	Fajita Pasta (Page 159)	15.20	55.6	8.78	2.66	363
	3 cups raw vegetable salad	6.00	15	0	6	75
	2 tablespoons vinegar	0.00	0	0	0	58
	1 ½ tablespoons oil	0.00	0	6.75	0	60

		Protein	Carbs	Fat	Fiber	Calories
Snack	Black-Eyed Pea Salad (Page 255)	6.10	21.3	2.25	1.4	130
	1 serving fruit	0.00	15	0	2	60
	1 tablespoon peanut butter	4.00	3.5	8	0.5	95.5
Quick Snack	3 cups raw vegetables	6.00	15	0	12	75
	3 tablespoons light salad dressing	0.00	10.5	9	0	120
	Totals	81.66	275.70	61.78	40.56	2,003.50

2,000-Calorie Meal Plans: Friday

		Protein	Carbs	Fat	Fiber	Calories
Breakfast	Breakfast Frittata (Page 234)	15.20	17.65	13.45	1	253
	¾ cup of light yogurt	6.00	20	0	0	110
	1 serving fruit	0.00	15	0	3	60
Lunch	Tangy Peach and Whole Grain Salad ½ (Page 29)	11.90	57	16.3	3	423
	2 cups raw leafy greens	4.00	10	0	8	50
	½ serving fruit	0.00	7.5	0	1.5	30

(Continued)

		Protein	Carbs	Fat	Fiber	Calories
Dinner	Parsnips and Pork Loin (Page 252)	9.79	62	4.9	4.49	332
	2 ounces pork loin	14.80	0	2	0	81
	1 ½ cups cooked vegetables	6.00	15	0	12	75
Snack	Greek Salad (Page 250)	3.50	32	4	1	179
	1 ounce almonds	6.00	0	14	3.3	164
Quick Snack	2 cups raw celery	4	10	0	8	50
	1 tablespoon peanut butter	4.00	3.5	8	0.5	95.5
	2 tablespoons dried fruit	0.00	15	0	3	60
	Totals	85.19	272.15	62.65	50.29	1,992.50

2,000-Calorie Meal Plans: Saturday

		Protein	Carbs	Fat	Fiber	Calories
Breakfast	Heirloom Benedict (Page 159)	13.20	30.5	14.1	7.8	302
	1 serving fruit	0.00	15	0	3	60
	1 cup nonfat milk	8.00	12	1	0	100
Lunch	Satisfaction Solution Salad (Page 30)	11.45	32.5	9.6	4.1	262

		Protein	Carbs	Fat	Fiber	Calories
	White Beans and Pesto, 2 (Page 258)	9.00	24	2	1.2	154
	1 serving fruit	0.00	15	0	3	60
	Black olives, 8	0.40	2.79	4.3	1.4	48
Dinner	Baked Crispy Chicken (Page 190)	20.75	25.6	9.3	0.09	270
	Pumpkin Pancakes (Page 235)	5.98	24.1	1.7	4.35	136
	Light maple syrup, 2 tablespoons	0.00	13.5	0	0.5	52
	½ cup cooked vegetables	2.00	5	0	4	25
	½ serving fruit	0.00	7.5	0	1.5	30
Snack	Tofu Dip, 2 servings (Page 256)	6.88	4.48	2	0.06	82
	3 cups raw vegetables	6.00	15	0	10	75
	1 serving fruit	0.00	15	0	3	60
Quick Snack	¼ cup dried fruit	0.00	30	0	6	120
	1 ounce almonds	6.00	0	14	3.3	164
	Totals	89.66	271.97	57.98	53.30	2,000.00

2,200-Calorie Meal Plans: Sunday

		Protein	Carbs	Fat	Fiber	Calories
Breakfast	Breakfast Smoothie	10.20	34.4	5.59	3.8	229
	1 slice whole grain toast	3.50	11.3	1.1	1.9	69
	1 tablespoon peanut butter	4.00	3.5	8	0.5	95.5
	½ cup milk	3.50	6	0	0	50
Lunch	Shrimp Taco, 2 (Page 15)	23.50	38.6	3.5	3	281
	4 tablespoons avocado	0.00	0	10	6	90
	1 ½ cups salad	3.00	7.5	0	4.5	39.5
	1 tablespoon vinegar	0.00	0	0	0	25
	Cilantro Soup (Page 256)	1.00	35.1	0.59	1.44	150
Dinner	Asian Flank Steak (Page 245)	12.20	5.9	13	0.15	190
	Cucumber Salad, 1 ½ servings (Page 244)	2.60	16.5	5.6	0.6	124.5
	One sandwich thin-two halves, whole wheat	5.00	21	1	6	100
	1 serving fruit	0.00	15	0	3	60
	Greek yogurt, plain, ½ cup	7.50	3	0	0	40
	1 tablespoon honey	0.00	17	0	0	60

		Protein	Carbs	Fat	Fiber	Calories
Snack	Bean Slaw (Page 78)	6.23	19.8	7.7	2.28	174
	1 cup nonfat milk	8.00	12	4	0	100
	1 serving fruit	0.00	15	0	3	60
Quick Snack	Corn and Avocado Dip (Page 255)	3.90	16.3	8.05	2	152
	2 cups raw vegetables	4.00	10	0	8	50
	1 serving fruit	0.00	15	0	3	60
	Totals	98.13	302.90	68.13	49.17	2,199.50

2,200-Calorie Meal Plans: Monday

		Protein	Carbs	Fat	Fiber	Calories
Breakfast	Baked Oatmeal Casserole (Page 246)	7.80	50.4	8.1	2.26	307
	½ serving fruit	0.00	7.5	0	1.5	30
	½ cup nonfat milk	4.00	6	0.5	0	50
Lunch	Brie and Pear Sandwich (Page 14)	21.90	35	10.9	7.1	327
	Cauliflower Tabbouleh (Page 77)	2.30	6.97	6.79	0.95	98
	Greek yogurt, plain, 1 cup	15.00	6	0	0	80

(Continued)

		Protein	Carbs	Fat	Fiber	Calories
	1 tablespoon honey	0.00	17	0	0	60
	½ serving fruit	0.00	7.5	0	1.5	30
Dinner	Smoky Sweet Corn Risotto (Page 189)	4.80	59.2	10	3.79	348
	1 ½ cups cooked vegetables	6.00	12.5	0	12	75
	1 tablespoon butter/ margarine	0.00	0	11.5	0	102
Snack	Hearts of Palm Salad (Page 250)	3.90	9.1	14.5	2.39	183
	1 ½ servings fruit	0.00	22.5	0	3	90
	1 cup nonfat milk	8.00	12	1	0	100
Quick Snack	Tofu Dip, 3 servings (Page 256)	10.30	6.72	3.04	0.09	123
	3 cups raw vegetables	6.00	15	0	12	75
	2 servings fruit	0.00	30	0	6	120
	Totals	90.00	303.39	66.34	52.58	2,198.00

2,200-Calorie Meal Plans: Tuesday

		Protein	Carbs	Fat	Fiber	Calories
Breakfast	Figgy Quinoa Pudding (Page 44)	6.40	32.9	2.6	2.15	181

		Protein	Carbs	Fat	Fiber	Calories
	1 serving fruit	0.00	15	0	0	60
	1 cup nonfat milk	8.00	12	1	0	100
Lunch	Gazpacho, 2 servings (Page 77)	5.52	32.8	9.9	3.6	242
	Sweet Mexican Salad (Page 256)	10.00	42.8	0.92	3.3	220
	4 tablespoons avocado	0.00	0	10	6	90
Dinner	Baked Breaded Salmon (Page 246)	23.50	17.7	8.2	0.1	239
	Walnut Pesto (Page 171)	3.00	4.1	16.1	1.59	173
	2 cups cooked vegetables	8.00	20	0	16	100
	⅔ cup cooked brown rice	6.00	30	2		160
	½ serving fruit	0.00	7.5	0	1.5	30
Snack	Black Bean Dip (Page 201)	4.90	14.7	0.31	1.1	81
	3 cups raw vegetables	6.00	15	0	12	75
	1 serving fruit	0.00	15	0	3	60

(Continued)

		Protein	Carbs	Fat	Fiber	Calories
Quick Snack	1 ounce peanuts	6.70	6.1	14	3.25	166
	4 tablespoons dried fruit	0.00	30	0	6	120
	1 cup nonfat milk	8.00	12	1	0	100
	Totals	96.02	307.60	66.03	59.59	2,197.00

2,200-Calorie Meal Plans: Wednesday

		Protein	Carbs	Fat	Fiber	Calories
Breakfast	Fruited Oatmeal (Page 148)	8.30	32.2	13.3	2.48	282
	1 serving fruit (Page 150)	0.00	15	0	3	60
	1 cup nonfat milk	8.00	12	1	0	100
Lunch	Black Bean and Wheat Berry Salad (Page 70)	20.00	40	13.5	3.6	363
	3 cups mixed greens	6.00	15	0	6	75
	1 serving fruit	0.00	15	0	3	60
	1 tablespoon peanut butter	4.00	3.5	8	0.5	95.5
Dinner	Cajun Jambalaya (Page 42)	18.30	60.8	8.18	1.9	390
	1 ½ cups cooked vegetables	6.00	15	0	12	75

		Protein	Carbs	Fat	Fiber	Calories
Snack	Tortilla Salad (Page 257)	5.90	23.9	3.6	1.96	152
	Greek yogurt, plain, ½ cup	7.00	3	0	0	40
	1 tablespoon honey	0.00	17	0	0	60
Quick Snack	⅓ cup dried fruit	0.00	45	0	6	180
	1 ½ ounces almonds	9.00	0	21	4.9	246
	Totals	92.50	297.40	68.58	45.34	2,178.50

2,200-Calorie Meal Plans: Thursday

		Protein	Carbs	Fat	Fiber	Calories
Breakfast	Fruited Granola (Page 150)	9.70	54.9	5.1	5	305
	½ serving fruit	0.00	7.5	0	1.5	30
Lunch	Satisfaction Solution Wrap (Page 254)	18.10	26.8	20.9	8.7	368
	Watermelon Salad, 2 servings (Page 258)	1.56	27.6	1	0.8	124
	Greek yogurt, plain, 1cup	15.00	6	0	0	80
	1 tablespoon honey	0.00	17	0	0	60

(Continued)

		Protein	Carbs	Fat	Fiber	Calories
Dinner	Fajita Pasta (Page 159)	15.20	55.6	8.78	2.66	363
	3 cups raw vegetable salad	6.00	15	0	6	75
	2 tablespoons vinegar	0.00	0	0	0	58
	1 ½ tablespoons oil	0.00	0	6.75	0	60
Snack	Black-Eyed Pea Salad (Page 255)	6.10	21.3	2.25	1.4	130
	¼ cup low-fat cottage cheese	7.00	0	3	0	45
	2 servings fruit	0.00	30	0	4	120
	1 tablespoon peanut butter	4.00	3.5	8	0.5	95.5
Quick Snack	3 cups raw vegetables	6.00	15	0	12	75
	3 tablespoons light salad dressing	0.00	10.5	9	0	120
	1 cup nonfat milk	8.00	12	1	0	100
	Totals	96.66	302.70	65.78	42.56	2,208.50

2,200-Calorie Meal Plans: Friday

		Protein	Carbs	Fat	Fiber	Calories
Breakfast	Breakfast Frittata (Page 234)	15.20	17.65	13.45	1	253

		Protein	Carbs	Fat	Fiber	Calories
	¾ cup of Light yogurt	6.00	20	0	0	110
	½ – ¾ cup 100% juice	0.00	15	0	3	60
	½ serving Fruit	0.00	7.5	0	1.5	30
Lunch	Tangy Peach and Whole Grain Salad 1 ½ servings (Page 29)	11.90	57	16.3	3	423
	2 cups raw leafy greens	4.00	10	0	8	50
	½ serving Fruit	0.00	7.5	0	1.5	30
Dinner	Parsnips (and Pork Loin)	9.79	62	4.9	4.49	332
	2 ounces pork loin	14.80	0	2	0	81
	1 ½ cups cooked vegetables	6.00	15	0	12	75
Snack	Greek Salad (Page 232)	3.50	32	4	1	179
	1 ounce almonds	6.00	0	14	3.3	164
	1 cup nonfat milk	8.00	12	1	0	100
Quick Snack	2 cups raw celery	4	10	0	8	50
	2 tablespoons peanut butter	8.00	7	16	1	191.1
	3 tablespoons dried fruit	0.00	22.5	0	6	90
	Totals	97.19	295.15	71.65	53.79	2,218.10

2,200-Calorie Meal Plans: Saturday

		Protein	Carbs	Fat	Fiber	Calories
Breakfast	Heirloom Benedict (Page 147)	13.20	30.5	14.1	7.8	302
	1 serving fruit	0.00	15	0	3	60
	1 cup nonfat milk	8.00	12	1	0	100
Lunch	Satisfaction Solution Salad (Page 33)	11.45	32.5	9.6	4.1	262
	White Beans and Pesto, 2 servings (Page 240)	9.00	24	2	1.2	154
	1 serving fruit	0.00	15	0	3	60
	Black olives, 12	0.60	4.1	6.45	2.1	72
Dinner	Baked Crispy Chicken (Page 175)	20.75	25.6	9.3	0.09	270
	Pumpkin Pancakes (Page 217)	5.98	24.1	1.7	4.35	136
	Light maple syrup, 2 tablespoons	0.00	13.5	0	0.5	52
	½ cup cooked vegetables	2.00	5	0	4	25
	½ serving fruit	0.00	7.5	0	1.5	30

		Protein	Carbs	Fat	Fiber	Calories
Snack	Tofu Dip, 2 servings (Page 238)	6.88	4.48	2	0.06	82
	2 cups raw vegetables	4.00	10	0	8	50
	½ cup milk	4.00	6	0.5	0	50
	2 servings fruit	0.00	30	0	6	120
Quick Snack	¼ cup dried fruit	0.00	30	0	6	120
	1 ounce almonds	6.00	0	14	3.3	164
	¼ cup low-fat cottage cheese	7.00	0	3	0	45
	1 serving fruit	0.00	15	0	3	60
	Totals	98.86	304.28	63.63	58.00	2,214.00

2,500-Calorie Meal Plans: Sunday

		Protein	Carbs	Fat	Fiber	Calories
Breakfast	Breakfast Smoothie 1½ servings (Page 247)	15.30	51.6	8.3	5.7	343.5
	1 slice whole grain toast	3.50	11.3	1.1	1.9	69
	1½ tablespoons peanut butter	6.00	5.25	12	0.75	143.25
	½ serving fruit	0.00	7.5	0	1.5	30

(Continued)

		Protein	Carbs	Fat	Fiber	Calories
Lunch	Shrimp Tacos, 2 (Page 15)	23.50	38.6	3.5	3	281
	4 tablespoons avocado	0.00	0	10	6	90
	1 ½ cups salad	3.00	7.5	0	4.5	39.5
	Cilantro Soup (Page 256)	1.00	35.1	0.59	1.44	150
Dinner	Asian Flank Steak (Page 245)	12.20	5.9	13	0.15	190
	Cucumber Salad, 1 ½ servings (Page 244)	2.60	16.5	5.6	0.6	124.5
	One sandwich thin-two halves, whole wheat	5.00	21	1	6	100
	1 serving fruit	0.00	15	0	3	60
	Greek yogurt, plain, ½ cup	7.50	3	0	0	40
	1 tablespoon honey	0.00	17	0	0	60
Snack	Bean Slaw (Page 78)	6.23	19.8	7.7	2.28	174
	1 cup nonfat milk	8.00	12	4	0	100
	1 serving fruit	0.00	15	0	3	60
Quick Snack	Corn and Avocado Dip, 2 servings (Page 255)	7.80	32.6	16.1	4	304

	Protein	Carbs	Fat	Fiber	Calories
3 cups raw vegetables	6.00	15	0	12	75
1 serving fruit	0.00	15	0	3	60
Totals	107.63	344.65	82.89	58.82	2,483.75

2,500-Calorie Meal Plans: Monday

		Protein	Carbs	Fat	Fiber	Calories
Breakfast	Baked Oatmeal Casserole (Page 246)	7.80	50.4	8.1	2.26	307
	1 serving fruit	0.00	15	0	3	60
	1 cup nonfat milk	8.00	12	1	0	100
Lunch	Brie and Pear Sandwich (Page 14)	21.90	35	10.9	7.1	327
	Cauliflower Tabbouleh (Page 77)	2.30	6.97	6.79	0.95	98
	Greek yogurt, plain, 1 cup	15.00	6	0	0	80
	1 tablespoon honey	0.00	17	0	0	60
	½ serving fruit	0.00	7.5	0	1.5	30
Dinner	Smoky Sweet Corn Risotto (Page 189)	4.80	59.2	10	3.79	348
	1 ½ cups cooked vegetables	6.00	12.5	0	12	75

(Continued)

		Protein	Carbs	Fat	Fiber	Calories
	1 ½ tablespoons butter/ margarine	0.00	0	17.3	0	153
Snack	Hearts of Palm Salad, 1 ½ servings (Page 250)	4.68	13.65	21.8	3.5	274.5
	2 servings fruit	0.00	30	0	6	120
	1 cup nonfat milk	8.00	12	1	0	100
Quick Snack	Tofu Dip, 3 servings (Page 256)	10.30	6.7	3	0.09	123
	3 cups raw vegetables	6.00	15	0	12	75
	6 tablespoons dried fruit	0.00	45	0	6	180
	Totals	94.78	343.92	79.80	58.19	2,510.50

2,500-Calorie Meal Plans: Tuesday

		Protein	Carbs	Fat	Fiber	Calories
Breakfast	Figgy Quinoa Pudding, 2 servings (Page 44)	12.80	65.8	5.2	4.3	362
	½ serving fruit	0.00	7.5	0	0	30
	1 tablespoon peanut butter	4.00	3.5	8	0.5	95.5
	½ cup nonfat milk	4.00	6	0.5	0	50

		Protein	Carbs	Fat	Fiber	Calories
Lunch	Gazpacho, 2 servings (Page 77)	5.52	32.8	9.9	3.6	242
	Sweet Mexican Salad (Page 256)	10.00	42.8	0.92	3.3	220
	4 tablespoons avocado	0.00	0	10	6	90
Dinner	Baked Breaded Salmon, 1 ½ servings (Page 246)	35.20	26.5	12	0.1	358.5
	Walnut Pesto, 1 ½ servings (Page 171)	4.50	6.15	24.15	1.3	259.5
	2 cups cooked vegetables	8.00	20	0	16	100
	½ cup cooked brown rice	2.30	22.9	0.8	1.8	109
Snack	Black Bean Dip, 2 servings (Page 201)	9.80	29.4	0.62	2.2	162
	3 cups raw vegetables	6.00	15	0	12	75
	1 serving fruit	0.00	15	0	3	60
Quick Snack	¼ cup low-fat-cottage cheese	7.00	0	3	0	45
	½ cup dried fruit	0.00	60	0	8	240
	Totals	109.12	353.35	75.09	62.10	2,498.50

2,500-Calorie Meal Plans: Wednesday

		Protein	Carbs	Fat	Fiber	Calories
Breakfast	Fruited Oatmeal, 1 ½ servings (Page 148)	12.45	48.3	19.9	3.7	423
	1 serving fruit	0.00	15	0	3	60
	1 cup nonfat milk	8.00	12	1	0	100
Lunch	Black Bean and Wheat Berry Salad (Page 70)	20.00	40	13.5	3.6	363
	3 cups mixed greens	6.00	15	0	6	75
	1 serving fruit	0.00	15	0	3	60
	1 tablespoon peanut butter	4.00	3.5	8	0.5	95.5
Dinner	Cajun Jambalaya (Page 42)	18.30	60.8	8.18	1.9	390
	1 ½ cups cooked vegetables	6.00	15	0	12	75
Snack	Tortilla Salad (Page 257)	5.90	23.9	3.6	1.96	152
	Greek yogurt, plain, 1 cup	17.00	6	0	0	80
	1 tablespoon honey	0.00	17	0	0	60
	1 serving fruit	0.00	15	0	3	60

		Protein	Carbs	Fat	Fiber	Calories
Quick Snack	½ cup dried fruit	0.00	60	0	8	240
	1 ½ ounces almonds	9.00	0	21	4.9	246
	Totals	106.65	346.50	75.18	51.56	2,479.50

2,500-Calorie Meal Plans: Thursday

		Protein	Carbs	Fat	Fiber	Calories
Breakfast	Fruited Granola (Page 150)	9.70	54.9	5.1	5	305
	1 serving fruit	0.00	15	0	3	60
Lunch	Satisfaction Solution Wrap (Page 254)	18.10	26.8	20.9	8.7	368
	Watermelon Salad, 2 servings (Page 258)	1.56	27.6	1	0.8	124
	Greek Yogurt, plain, 1cup	15.00	6	0	0	80
	1 tablespoon honey	0.00	17	0	0	60
Dinner	Fajita Pasta (Page 159)	15.20	55.6	8.78	2.66	363
	3 cups raw vegetable salad	6.00	15	0	6	75
	2 tablespoons vinegar	0.00	0	0	0	58

(Continued)

		Protein	Carbs	Fat	Fiber	Calories
	1 ½ tablespoons oil	0.00	0	6.75	0	60
	½ serving fruit	0.00	7.5	0	1.5	30
Snack	Black-Eyed Pea Salad, 2 servings (Page 255)	12.20	42.6	4.5	2.8	260
	¼ cup low-fat cottage cheese	7.00	0	3	0	45
	1 serving fruit	0.00	15	0	2	60
	1 tablespoon peanut butter	4.00	3.5	8	0.5	95.5
Quick Snack	3 cups raw vegetables	6.00	15	0	12	75
	2 tablespoons light salad dressing	0.00	7	6	0	80
	1 cup nonfat milk	8.00	12	1	0	100
	1 ounce almonds	6.00	0	14	3.3	164
	1 serving fruit	0.00	15	0	3	60
	Totals	108.76	335.50	79.03	51.26	2,522.50

2,500-Calorie Meal Plans: Friday

		Protein	Carbs	Fat	Fiber	Calories
Breakfast	Breakfast Frittata, 1 ½ servings (Page 234)	22.80	26.4	20.1	1.5	379.5

		Protein	Carbs	Fat	Fiber	Calories
	light yogurt	6.00	20	0	0	110
	½ – ¾ cup 100% juice	0.00	15	0	3	60
	1 serving fruit	0.00	15	0	3	60
Lunch	Tangy Peach and Whole Grain Salad, 1 ½ servings (Page 29)	11.90	57	16.3	3	423
	2 cups raw leafy greens	4.00	10	0	8	50
	½ serving fruit	0.00	7.5	0	1.5	30
Dinner	Parsnips and Pork Loin (Page 252)	9.79	62	4.9	4.49	332
	2 ounces pork loin	14.80	0	2	0	81
	1 ½ cups cooked vegetables	6.00	15	0	12	75
Snack	Greek Salad (Page 250)	3.50	32	4	1	179
	1 ounce almonds	6.00	0	14	3.3	164
	1 cup nonfat milk	8.00	12	1	0	100
	1 serving fruit	0.00	15	0	3	60
Quick Snack	3 cups raw celery	6	15	0	12	75
	2 tablespoons peanut butter	8.00	7	16	1	191.1

(Continued)

	Protein	Carbs	Fat	Fiber	Calories
4 tablespoons dried fruit	0.00	30	0	8	120
Totals	106.79	338.90	78.30	64.79	2,489.60

2,500-Calorie Meal Plans: Saturday

		Protein	Carbs	Fat	Fiber	Calories
Breakfast	Heirloom Benedict (Page 159)	13.20	30.5	14.1	7.8	302
	1 serving fruit	0.00	15	0	3	60
	1 tablespoon peanut butter	4.00	3.5	8	0.5	95.5
	½ cup nonfat milk	4.00	6	0.5	0	50
	light yogurt	6.00	20	0	0	110
Lunch	Satisfaction Solution Salad (Page 30)	11.45	32.5	9.6	4.1	262
	White Beans and Pesto, 2 servings (Page 258)	9.00	24	2	1.2	154
	1 serving fruit	0.00	15	0	3	60
	Black olives, 12	0.60	4.1	6.45	2.1	72
Dinner	Baked Crispy Chicken (Page 190)	20.75	25.6	9.3	0.09	270
	Pumpkin Pancakes (Page 235)	5.98	24.1	1.7	4.35	136

		Protein	Carbs	Fat	Fiber	Calories
	Light maple syrup, 2 tablespoons	0.00	13.5	0	0.5	52
	1 cup cooked vegetables	4.00	10	0	8	50
	½ tablespoon butter/ margarine	0.00	0	5.75	0	51
	½ serving fruit	0.00	7.5	0	1.5	30
Snack	Tofu Dip, 3 servings (Page 256)	10.30	6.7	3	0.09	123
	3 cups raw vegetables	6.00	15	0	12	75
	2 servings fruit	0.00	30	0	6	120
	1 ounce almonds	6.00	0	14	3.3	164
Quick Snack	¼ cup dried fruit	0.00	30	0	6	120
	2 servings fruit	0.00	30	0	6	120
	¼ cup low-fat cottage cheese	7.00	0	3	0	45
	Totals	108.28	343.00	77.38	69.53	2,521.50

Satisfaction Solution: Eat Five Times a Day

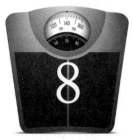

Learn Why It's Important to Eat Small Meals Several Times a Day

The first key to losing weight: Eat! It might seem counterintuitive, but fueling your body every few hours is exactly what you need to keep your metabolism revving and to lose weight while feeling satisfied.

Start with Breakfast

Research consistently shows that eating breakfast helps people lose weight. In fact, people who skip breakfast are more likely to be obese [4]. Breakfast even helps you perform better when you get to work [5].

> Research consistently shows that eating breakfast helps people lose weight.

Your blood sugar levels are low in the morning after up to twelve hours without food. Eating a healthy breakfast gives you physical and mental energy to get through the morning. When you don't have breakfast, you're likely to feel tired and irritable, and you're more likely to go overboard at lunchtime [6].

Plain and simple: People who are successful at losing weight and keeping it off eat breakfast. Among almost three thousand people registered with the National Weight Control Registry, 78 percent say they eat breakfast every day [7].

Another study that followed the eating patterns of more than two thousand adolescents over five years found that those who ate breakfast more often had lower body weights [8].

Some healthy breakfast options: peanut butter and banana slices on whole wheat toast with a glass of milk, or oatmeal made with nonfat milk and topped with dried fruit and chopped walnuts [9].

Then Eat About Every Three Hours

It takes your stomach about three or four hours to empty, and then it's time to eat again [10]. However, many people try to push that timeframe and go longer without eating, says Bonnie Taub-Dix, RD, owner of BTD Nutrition Consultants in New York and Long Island and author of Read It Before You Eat It [11].

We all know that if we let ourselves get too hungry we're likely to inhale any food we can get our hands on, whether it's the healthy steak tacos planned for dinner or the ready-to-eat cookie dough that's sitting in the freezer [11].

> Eating at around the same time every day trains your body to expect food when it's time to eat and helps you avoid feeling hungry when it's not time to eat.

A big reason that happens is blood sugar, Taub-Dix says. When your blood sugar becomes too low because it's been too long since you last ate, you'll feel shaky, dizzy, weak, and irritable, she says. "You're also really likely to make poor food choices when your blood sugar is dropping like that," she says. Low blood sugar literally makes it harder for you to think clearly [11]. So you run to the snack machine at work or stop at the first McDonald's.

A recent study, recounted in an article in the British Journal of Nutrition, by Miriam Clegg and Amir Shafat, demonstrated that high-fat breakfasts can actually lead to more food intake later, while a low-fat, high-fiber breakfast increased fullness and decreased appetite later in the day [12].

Also, eating at around the same time every day trains your body to expect food when it's time to eat and helps you avoid feeling hungry when it's not time to eat. "Some people don't like to be held to a schedule, but spontaneity can be risky," Taub-Dix says [11].

In addition, eating this way may burn more calories, since digesting food burns calories for a short amount of time [13].

What Works for Me

Jennifer Doyle, a school administrator in Rochester, NY

From the time I was in middle school, I never ate breakfast. I went through every morning on a completely empty stomach and ate my first meal at around noon.

Then, five years ago, I found myself at 180 pounds and very unhappy. My mornings may have been sparse on food, but when I did start eating I practically didn't stop. I ate big meals, fatty meals, fried foods, and snacks all the time. Whenever I felt hungry I'd grab a bag of chips or a candy bar. I was also in terrible physical shape. I literally felt as if I wasn't fit enough to work out. When I tried exercise, I felt tired and just gross.

The epiphany that I needed to do something came when I watched the very first *Biggest Loser*. A woman on the show was my height and weight, and she looked awful. I happened to have a doctor's appointment soon after seeing the show, and my cholesterol was extremely high. I realized it was time to change.

I chose a low-carb diet because some friends of mine had lost a significant amount of weight eating that way. But I knew before I started that if I was going to do this, I was going to have to get reacquainted with a meal that I hadn't eaten in more than two decades: breakfast. My friends who had lost weight had already warned me that breakfast is an essential part of weight loss. Plus, the diet I started had breakfasts built into the plan.

Once I started eating breakfast and eating healthier all day long, I naturally fell into a pattern where I ate healthy snacks or meals every few hours. Some days I would eat dinner pretty early, around 3:30 or 4 p.m. when I got home from work. Then I had a snack before bed. Eating this way helped satisfy my hunger as I lost weight.

Since then, breakfast has been a regular part of my day, and I feel so much better eating it. I know if I go too long before eating breakfast in the morning I'll be really hungry and may not make the best food choices. On weekends when I can sleep in, I get up at 7 a.m. to let my dogs outside. Before heading back to bed I'll have a quick snack, such as yogurt and a piece of fruit.

Eating this way was a real paradigm shift for me. In the past I ate and drank to my heart's content without thinking about the consequences. Food was the centerpiece of my days and nights. Now I've learned to step back and ask myself, "Do I really need to eat or drink this right now?" I had been living to eat, but now I'm eating to live.

You'll have to look at your daily schedule to figure out what works for you, Taub-Dix says. For the average person, an ideal meal pattern might be: breakfast, lunch, snack, dinner, and a snack, she says. But if you're an early riser who eats breakfast at 6 a.m., waiting until noon to eat is only going to set you up to blow your diet. If that's the case for you, plan a midmorning snack and get rid of the late night snack [11].

Here are three examples of how you might plan your day:

8 a.m. Breakfast

11 a.m. Lunch

2 p.m. Snack

5 p.m. Dinner

8 p.m. Snack

Or

6 a.m. Breakfast

9 a.m. Midmorning Snack

12 p.m. Lunch

3 p.m. Afternoon Snack

6 p.m. Dinner

Or

6 a.m. Breakfast

9 a.m. Midmorning Snack

12 p.m. Lunch

3 p.m. Pre-exercise Snack

4 p.m. Exercise

5 p.m. Post-exercise Snack

6 p.m. Dinner

Portions are also key. Aim to get about 150 calories from each snack and 400 calories from each meal depending on your calorie needs.

Make Every Meal and Snack High Quality

Some people say that the more times you eat during the day, the more opportunities you have for overeating. Instead, think of it as giving yourself more opportunities to eat well and stave off hunger, Taub-Dix says [11].

It's obvious that reaching for junk food five times a day is only going to undermine your goals. It's also going to make you hungrier than you would be if you aim for quality foods that fill you up [11].

For example, choosing a whole-grain cereal in the morning is healthier because it's full of fiber. In a study of thirty-two men and women, those who ate a breakfast cereal that included 26 grams of insoluble fiber ate fewer calories at breakfast and at lunch compared to those who ate cereal with only 1 gram of fiber. Those who ate the high-fiber cereal also had lower blood sugar levels before and after lunch [14].

In the next chapter you'll learn that combining foods, such as protein and carbohydrates, is the best way to keep your blood sugar levels stable and your hunger under control. Be sure your meals and snacks are balanced and nutritious. A typical day might include whole-grain cereal with nonfat milk and orange juice with pulp for breakfast, baby carrots and sliced jicama dipped in seasoned Greek yogurt for a snack, a whole-wheat wrap filled with veggies and sliced turkey and a banana for lunch, part-skim cheese with whole-wheat crackers for another snack, and broiled fish, steamed asparagus and couscous for dinner, with grilled pineapple for dessert [11].

Don't Fudge It

Nutritionists know that some of us have become masters at ignoring hunger signals. We're notorious for wanting to lose weight and wanting to lose it now, so we think skipping meals or going on fad diets will get us to our unrealistic goals even faster.

When the stomach starts to rumble between meals, we might reach for a diet soda or a cup of coffee to try to quiet it. But that's a problem, says Lisa Bunce, RD, owner of Back to Basics Nutrition Consulting in Redding, Conn., who developed the My Lil'Coach app (available at www.mylilcoach.com) [10].

"If it's true physical hunger, it's time for an apple or some nuts,"

Bunce says [10].

What's most important is honoring your body and giving it what it needs—not trying to make your body change on an impossible schedule. Listen to your body's messages of feeling hungry, plan ahead to eat the right foods when it's time, and be patient about the results. If you keep it up, you'll see your body change. Think of all the years it took to add the weight on; it is going to take time to get rid of those unhealthy habits and lose the weight.

Dietitian's Diary

Feeling Good About Yourself

There is a misconception that we are strong if we can lose weight and weak if we are overweight. In truth, losing weight is a learning process about ourselves, emotionally and physically. It takes time to learn about food and discover new foods you enjoy eating. Be patient with yourself; the weight did not end up on your thighs overnight, so sustainable weight loss will not happen overnight either.

You'll find hope in your perseverance. In fact, recent studies show that maintaining weight loss can result in a definite and positive shift in self-perception. As Dr. Eleni Epiphaniou pointed out in the article "Successful Weight Loss Maintenance and a Shift in Identity from Restriction to a New Liberated Self," in the January 2010 edition of the Journal of Health Psychology, "a previously restrained self (becomes) a liberated individual, regarding their social interactions, dietary habits, emotional regulation and self-appraisal." (Dr. Epiphaniou is a researcher at King's College, London, where she focuses on behavior change, and in particular how people's experiences, beliefs, and expectations influence the endorsement of a healthy or unhealthy behavior.) [15].

We encourage you to keep a journal of your weight-loss challenges and successes. Then you'll see, in black and white, how strong you really are. (Go back to Chapter 7 to review directions for putting your journal together.)

Fad Diets

The definition of "fad" is: "practice or interest followed for a time with exaggerated zeal" (Merriam Webster). To me, "for a time" is the operative phrase when it comes to fad diets. It seems, based on the popularity of fad diets in the last thirty years, we do not mind experimenting with our bodies for a short period of time as long as we see the numbers both on the scale and our waistlines go down. Some people have tried removing grains and fiber from their diet, some inject themselves with various hormones and/or supplements, some people have even tried harkening back to the Stone Age, eating like our ancestors.

The concept of ingesting out-of-the-ordinary items to affect our weight can be dated back to a myth about Cleopatra, the last pharaoh of Ancient Egypt [16]. The rumor in the scientific industry is that Cleopatra would swallow tapeworms to lose weight. For all we know, that could be the first recorded quick-weight-loss fad diet if it is ever proven. Throughout the centuries, and hundreds of fad diets later, the average weight of a person has increased dramatically, and one-third of the U.S. population is now considered obese [17]. It's not surprising then that we are so passionate about losing weight. We all have our reasons, ranging from doctor's orders to health goals to our personal vanity. The Satisfaction Solution is NOT a fad diet; it and is based on whole foods with a healthy balance of moderation and exercise.

Though you may see a decrease in your weight with a fad diet, there is a strong chance you may be negatively affecting your overall health in the process. Fad diets hang on one or several of the following principles and/or promises:

1. *Rapid weight loss.* For healthy sustainable weight loss, we should lose only one to two pounds a week. It is possible to lose more than that in the beginning, especially if you make several changes at once. For example, going from a sedentary lifestyle to exercising four days a week and substituting water for numerous sodas a day may increase your weight loss initially. You'll find, however, that your body will adapt to the new healthier lifestyle (since your body knows what is good for it), and your weight loss will level out to the healthy one to two pounds a week range.

2. *Elimination or restriction of entire food groups.* Each food group needs to be consumed for a biological and metabolic reason. Each group offers specific nutrients for our health and disease prevention. Even if you are able to stick to a radical diet's rules, such as low-to-no carbohydrates or eating nothing but cabbage soup, you will eventually be malnourished, and your body will react accordingly.

3. *Specific food combinations.* The process of eating your fruit first and your protein last is overthinking basic human nature. It all hits the stomach and becomes mixed together post-chew [18]. What you ate five minutes ago is being absorbed at the same time as what you are gnawing on now.

4. *Severely restricting calories.* For weight loss, calories consumed need to be fewer than calories spent. Thus, there needs to be a calorie deficit in the day to lose weight. As mentioned earlier, our body adapts to what we give it. With a healthy caloric deficit, the body will shed unnecessary weight. But, if we consume too few calories, in other words, the caloric deficit is too large, and the body goes into starvation mode. When this happens, the body doesn't start going after the fat we are trying to lose. Instead, our organs begin slowing down their functions and our metabolism slows. So, weight loss slows down, we are miserably hungry, we start to eat again, and the weight goes back on. There is also the risk of getting painful gallstones [19]. A good rule of thumb is that we need calories to burn calories.

5. *Rigid menus.* Simply put, these are not sustainable for anyone to live a healthy lifestyle.

6. *Lack of exercise.* We know we have to exercise for all over health and well-being. Exercise helps to raise our metabolism. It helps to build muscle to allow our bodies to function better and protect our organs. It helps strengthen our bones and tightens the skin around the parts of our body that used to be bigger. Any diet that claims you can lose weight without working out is not endorsing a healthy method of weight loss.

Recipes

To help you construct good, healthy breakfasts, use the grids below.

BREAKFAST OATMEAL GRID

Oatmeal, ½ cup cooked	Protein and Fat, 2 tablespoons	Flavor
Irish/steel cut oats	Almond	Brown sugar, 1 tablespoon
Scottish oats	Flaxseed meal, 2 tablespoons	Splenda brown sugar, 1 tablespoon
Rolled/old-fashioned oats	Pecans	Honey, 1 tablespoon
Instant, plain	Hazelnuts	Agave nectar, 1 tablespoon
	Walnuts	Cinnamon, to taste
	Pistachios	Calorie-free extracts, 1–2 teaspoons:
	Chestnuts	Almond
		Vanilla
		Orange
		Coconut
		Anise
		Brandy
		Rum
		Amaretto
		Strawberry
		Caramel

1. Cook oatmeal according to package directions. Use water method.
2. Stir in one option from the protein and one from the flavor column.

BREAKFAST QUINOA GRID   **Creates 6 servings, 1/3 cup each**

Quinoa	Milk	Flavoring	Dried Fruit
Amount: 1 cup	Amount: 1 ½ cups	Amount: 1–2 teaspoons each is defined as one serving)	Choose 4 servings below (each is defined as one serving)
Cream quinoa	Soy milk, light	Almond	Golden raisins, 2 tablespoons
Red quinoa	Soy milk, chocolate, light	Vanilla	Raisins, 2 tablespoons
Black quinoa	Rice milk	Orange	Cherries, 2 tablespoons
Quinoa flakes	1% milk	Coconut	Apricots, 4 whole, chopped
	Nonfat milk	Anise	Prunes, 3 whole, chopped
		Brandy	Blueberries, 2 tablespoons
		Rum	Cranberries, 2 tablespoons
		Amaretto	Apples, 4 rings, chopped
		Strawberry	Figs, 1 ½, chopped
		Caramel	Dates, 3 whole, chopped
		Mint	

1. Wash quinoa to remove any residue, called *saponin*, that can make quinoa taste bitter (remember this is a whole grain).

2. Combine 1 ½ cups of milk of your choosing and add 1 cup rinsed quinoa.

3. Bring to a boil.

4. Turn down heat and simmer for 15 minutes.

5. Remove from heat.

6. Let sit 5 minutes.

7. Stir in flavoring and dried fruit.

BREAKFAST GRANOLA GRID

Low-Fat Granola, 1/2 cup	Fresh Fruit, ½ cup	Protein and Fat, 2 tablespoons	Liquid, ½ -1 cup
		Almond milk	Almond
		Flaxseed meal	Soy milk, light
		Pecans	Soy milk, chocolate, light
		Hazelnuts	Rice milk
		Walnuts	1% milk
		Pistachios	Nonfat milk
		Chestnuts	Yogurt, plain
			Yogurt, Greek

Stir together one from each column and enjoy!

Satisfaction Solution: Combining Carbs with Protein or Fat

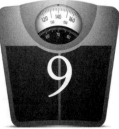

Learn Why It's Important to Combine Carbs with Healthy Proteins

Now that you know you're going to be eating five times today, what's on the menu?

Before you answer, we'll let you in on a little secret: losing weight while feeling full and satisfied means eating the right combination of foods.

It's not hard or complicated. You don't have to get out your calculator and brush up on your math skills. It's as simple as being sure that every meal and snack you eat has both carbohydrates and protein or fat. This could be the key to how you lose weight without feeling hungry.

"Americans tend to think in terms of one food item: a bowl of pasta or a piece of pizza," says Lisa Bunce. "But one food item doesn't fill us up" [1].

Although you'll lose weight any time you cut calories, studies have found that focusing on getting enough protein and fat helps people feel more satisfied while they lose weight. Protein not only helps people feel satisfied after one meal, but also the feeling of satiety lasts for twenty-four hours [2].

Studies also find that people who eat a moderate amount of carbohydrates along with higher amounts of protein are more likely to maintain weight loss for a year or more [2].

When you're eating fewer calories to lose weight, making this one change can make a big difference in the way you feel while you lose weight and how likely you are to be successful [1, 3].

Food Combining: Why It Works

When you eat a meal that has a combination of protein or fat and carbs, the food will leave your stomach more slowly, and you'll be able to get to your next meal without feeling hungry in the meantime [1].

151

Women in particular tend to grab crackers or cookies for a snack, but carbohydrates by themselves tend to break down very quickly and cause your blood sugar levels to rise and fall fast. Have a piece of candy when you're hungry, and your blood sugar will spike and crash like it's the stock market in 1929. When your blood sugar level falls fast, you're going to be ravenous for something else before it's time to eat again [3].

But when you pair a protein or a healthy fat with the carbohydrate, the food takes longer to break down. Your blood sugar rises more slowly and falls more slowly, so by the time you get hungry again it's lunchtime or dinnertime [3].

"I describe it as rolling hills," says Jessica Levinson, MS, RD, owner of Nutritioulicious, a nutrition counseling and consulting practice in New York City. The goal is to allow your blood sugar to rise and fall at a steady, slow rate throughout the day [3].

You're Probably Not Doing It, So ...

When Levinson's clients show her their food diaries for the first time, she often notices that they're not combining food the right way. They're eating crackers, pretzels, or a fruit as a snack in the afternoon, and by the time dinner rolls around, they're starving. And when they're starving, they're more likely to load up on rice or bread at dinner, or just plain eat a lot more than if they hadn't sat down at the dinner table feeling ravenous.

If you're female, you may not be getting enough protein overall. The National Health and Nutrition Examination Survey found that a significant number of women (particularly teenagers and older women) didn't get enough protein in their diet, which is about 17 percent to 21 percent of their calories. When it came to eating meat, only 37 percent of women age twenty and older got the minimum amount of recommended ounces of meat or meat alternatives in their diet, the survey found [4].

Even when you're being health conscious, it's easy to reach for carbs and forget about the protein. Levinson's clients think eating an apple or pretzels (which are low fat) is a healthy snack, but either option alone can cause your blood sugar to spike and then fall.

As you build a meal or snack, think about putting together at least three pieces of a puzzle, Bunce says: protein, a fiber-rich carbohydrate, and a fruit or vegetable. Instead of a big bowl of pasta, make it a little bowl of pasta with plenty of vegetables and a couple of small meatballs. Instead of a salad of only veggies, add some chickpeas and sliced turkey [1].

The All-Stars: Why Your Body Needs Them

You could say that carbs, protein, and fat are all-stars in your journey to lose weight without feeling hungry. Here are the roles each play in your body and why they're important for more than just filling you up.

Carbs

People tend to think carbs make them fat, but the truth is that anything you eat in excess will get stored as fat. And it's a lot easier to gorge on carbs than it is protein or fat. You're more likely to sit down in front of the television and eat hundreds of calories of chips, crackers, pretzels, or cereal than you are to munch on grilled chicken or salmon while you watch your favorite shows [3].

And with low-carb diets being the rage, it's easy to think that cutting carbs out of your diet will help you lose weight. But here's why you need to keep them on your plate: Carbs get broken down into glucose in your body, which is stored as energy. They contribute to physical energy as well as brain power. Eat too few carbs and you're going to be dragging during the day, physically and mentally [3].

Protein

Protein not only is the key to feeling full longer, but it also builds and repairs your body's tissues, helps create antibodies that fight infection, and helps to create enzymes and hormones [5].

Fat

Fat gives your body insulation, making you warm in the winter. "People who don't have enough fat in their diet are always cold," Levinson says. Fat also helps you absorb fat-soluble vitamins, such as vitamins A, D, E, and K, which help to give your body energy, make protein, heal, keep your bones strong, and help your vision [3].

Food-Combining Guidelines

As always, the carbs, protein, and fat you choose should be the most nutritious you can find. Not only will they nourish your body, but also they will add to your feeling of satisfaction after a meal. If you're eating lunch or dinner, fill half of your plate with vegetables, a quarter with lean protein, and the other quarter with healthy carbs, Levinson says [3].

Choosing Carbohydrates

A good quality carbohydrate (and one that's more filling and will keep your blood sugar levels stable) is made with whole grains. Choose brown rice, whole-wheat pasta, kasha, bulgur wheat, and tabbouleh [6]. When you're buying bread, rolls, pita, cereal, and crackers, check the ingredients list. If it's truly whole grain, it should say "100% whole grain" or "100% whole wheat" at the top of the ingredients list, Levinson says [3].

Healthy crackers, in particular, can be hard to find. A good place to look for a whole-grain cracker is in the natural food section of the supermarket. Levinson recommends choosing a cracker with 2 or 3 grams of fiber and less than 180 milligrams of sodium per serving [3].

Choosing Protein

Good protein sources include beans, legumes, peas, lentils, fish and seafood, chicken, turkey, eggs, beef, pork, veal, and lamb. Also, go for lean cuts of meat, and grill or bake your protein rather than frying it [7].

Choosing Fat

There are three types of healthy fats to aim for: monounsaturated (which include the fat found in avocado, canola oil, nuts, olive oil, peanut butter, and sesame seeds), polyunsaturated (which includes corn, safflower, soybean, sunflower, and cottonseed oil; walnuts; pumpkin and sunflower seeds; soft margarine; mayonnaise; and salad dressings), and omega-3 fatty acids (which include tofu, soybean products, walnuts, flaxseed oil, canola oil, and oil from fish like mackerel, salmon, sardines, rainbow trout, herring, and albacore tuna) [8].

 Even when you're being health conscious, it's easy to reach for carbs and forget about the protein.

Try to limit your intake of saturated fat (found in high-fat dairy products like ice cream and high-fat cheese, high-fat meats like ground beef and hot dogs, butter, lard, cream sauces, gravy, poultry skin, chocolate, palm oil, coconut oil, and fatback and salt pork) and trans fat (found in snacks like chips and baked goods; stick margarine; shortening; and some fast food, like French fries) [8].

If you think you can't lose weight because cutting calories leaves you too hungry, focus on food combining. You may find that it's easier to get to your next meal or snack without feeling starvation creeping in, and by the end of the day you'll have eaten fewer calories without even noticing.

Make a Satisfying Switcharoo

Take a look at your meals and snacks and see if you need to switch any of them with a more satisfying version [9].

Instead of eating ...	Have this instead ...
Just a cup of coffee for breakfast	A smoothie made with low-fat yogurt and frozen berries
White toast	Whole-grain toasted bread with one tablespoon of natural peanut or almond butter
A cereal bar	A bowl of whole-grain cereal with nonfat milk
A grapefruit	Oatmeal made with nonfat milk and mixed with raisins and walnuts, with half of a grapefruit on the side
Buttermilk waffles with syrup	A whole-wheat waffle topped with sliced banana and low-fat yogurt
A bagel	Half of a whole-grain bagel with almond butter and apple slices
An English muffin	A whole-grain English muffin with a slice of lean ham and low-fat Swiss cheese
A hard-boiled egg	A hard-boiled egg sliced and placed inside a whole-wheat pita with low-fat cheese
Scrambled eggs	An omelet made with veggies, such as peppers and spinach, with a sliced orange on the side
A deli sandwich made with white bread	Your own homemade sandwich using whole-grain bread, lean turkey, low-fat Swiss cheese, sliced tomatoes, sliced cucumbers, and lettuce leaves
A veggie salad	A veggie salad with beans, sliced turkey, or low-fat cheese
Ramen noodles or another pasta-heavy soup	Chicken noodle soup with a few whole-grain crackers
Two or three slices of pizza	One slice of veggie pizza with a generous veggie salad
A big bowl of pasta and sauce	A half-cup of pasta, veggies (such a peppers, eggplant, and squash), and a couple of small, lean meatballs
A 12-ounce steak with a baked potato	Three ounces of lean steak with a small baked sweet potato and steamed green beans
An apple	An apple with a tablespoon of natural peanut butter
Pretzels	Pretzels with part-skim string cheese
Soda	A milkshake made with nonfat milk, fruit, and ice
A bowl of berries	Greek yogurt mixed with whole-grain cereal, berries, and almonds

(Continued)

Instead of eating …	Have this instead …
A banana	A banana with a small handful of almonds or pistachios
Popcorn	Popcorn sprinkled with some parmesan cheese
A granola bar	A granola bar broken up and mixed into 6 ounces of low-fat yogurt
A candy bar	A square of dark chocolate with a cup of nonfat milk
Crackers	Whole-grain crackers with an ounce of part-skim cheese
A handful of raisins	A handful of trail mix with nuts, seeds, and dried fruit

What Works for Me

Jennette Fulda, author of *Half-Assed: A Weight-Loss Memoir* and *Chocolate & Vicodin: My Quest for Relief from the Headache that Wouldn't Go Away*, freelance writer and web designer in Chapel Hill, N.C. (For more information, go to JennetteFulda.com.)

I was a total dummy about nutrition before I lost nearly two hundred pounds. I know some women have dieted their whole lives and grew up knowing everything about carbs and calories and how many Weight Watchers points are in a box of Girl Scout Cookies. I was completely ignorant, so I was learning everything fresh. The briefest way to put it is that I learned my body runs best on lean meats, whole grains, and fruits and vegetables. You can't go too wrong with plants.

I started in January, which is the month gyms and diet programs are overrun with people making New Year's resolutions to lose weight. I was rather stereotypical in that manner, but the new year gave me the feeling of a fresh start.

I was also living with my younger brother and mother at the time, and I'd seen my brother have real success with a popular low-carb diet. I'd always thought diets were stupid fads that didn't work, but he was eating real food and not neon green shakes, so it looked like something I could do without suffering for the rest of my life.

My whole family changed our eating habits together. It was much easier to have their support. They weren't buying junk food that might tempt me when I opened the kitchen cabinets. It also helped to talk to them about everything I was learning about nutrition and cooking.

I had a very regular eating schedule, making sure to eat at least a snack every three hours. That way I was never ravenously hungry. I also tried to eat snacks with protein, like cheese sticks or pistachios, because protein keeps you fuller longer than carbs. Protein is also the macronutrient that takes the most energy to digest.

Besides that, I've learned that my body sometimes wants pleasure from food, though I don't technically need it. I was very hesitant to label myself as a food addict until I got a headache that lasted for over three years. When the pain was at its worst I started to use food as a drug, eating high-calorie, fatty foods like chocolate-covered pretzels so I could feel good, if only for five minutes. Trying to separate what my body needs from what it wants can be tricky, and I'm still figuring that out.

Building a Satisfying Salad

What better way to make a healthy lunch or dinner than to make a big salad? There's just one problem—if you don't build it with the right combination of veggies, protein, and fat, it won't hold you over to your next meal.

The key is to make greens and veggies the biggest part of your salad. They have the fewest number of calories and are full of fiber, which makes you feel full longer. Then add in a little fruit, a serving of protein, and a small amount of fat.

Step 1: Get your greens. Supermarkets and farmers' markets have a plethora of lettuces to choose from. Start with romaine, spinach, mixed greens, green- or red-leaf lettuce, Boston lettuce, escarole, arugula, iceberg, radicchio, or Napa cabbage [10].

Step 2: Mix in lots of veggies. Fill up your salad with bell peppers, peas, radishes, tomatoes, cucumbers, onion, water chestnuts, zucchini, beets, bean sprouts, artichoke hearts, bok choy, cauliflower, broccoli, carrots, corn, celery, or sugar snap peas [10].

Step 3: Sprinkle in some fruit. Go for dried fruit, such as raisins or dried cranberries, blueberries, or apricots. Or throw in sliced or whole fresh fruit, such as apple, melon, pear, strawberries, blueberries, Mandarin oranges, grapes, and grapefruit [10].

Step 4: Hit it with some protein. Now that you have the carbs, add beans, meat, seafood, or hard-boiled eggs to make it really satisfying. For beans, choose from black beans, edamame (soybeans), kidney beans, navy beans, or chickpeas. For meat, pick lean cuts of beef, chicken strips, or sliced ham or turkey (rolled and sliced). For seafood, go for cooked or canned salmon, tuna, or shrimp [10].

Step 5: Kick it up with healthy fat. For even more flavor and satisfaction, add in small amounts of low-fat cheese, such as feta, mozzarella, parmesan, cheddar, or blue cheese, or a small handful of nuts, such as almonds, pecans, walnuts, cashews, or peanuts. Another healthy fat option: sliced avocado or olives [10].

Step 6: Dress it well. You can add a store-bought dressing to your salad, but be sure it's not overloaded with saturated fat or sugar. Oil-based dressings tend to have healthier fats and are better options than creamy dressings like blue cheese, says Levinson [3].

But an even better option is to make your own healthy dressing. It's as simple as mixing together a tablespoon of extra-virgin olive oil and one or two tablespoons of vinegar, with salt and pepper to taste. If vinegar doesn't appeal to you, use fresh lemon, lime, or grapefruit juice [3, 11]. Add some more flavor with diced garlic, ginger, spices, or herbs.

Dietitian's Diary

The Fork Trick

Let's be honest: salad dressing is yummy! It makes dry lettuce easier to slide down the hatch and makes you crave the salad. But a serving of salad dressing can add more than three hundred calories to your oh-so-healthy salad. So I recommend the Fork Method.

Put or ask for dressing on the side. Then take your fork and dip it into the dressing. This will lightly coat the tip of the fork. Stab all your greens onto the fork and enjoy. You will get just enough flavor to enjoy, but not enough to defeat the purpose. When you are done with the salad, see how much dressing you have left!

Nothing to Fear

Carbohydrates. We cringe. We love them and we hate them; or at least, that is what the fad diets of the past have conjured up within us. I drool at the thought of warm Hawaiian bread coming out of the bread maker slathered in chilled butter as it cools the bread I am about to squish into my mouth. Then I cringe at the visual of the carbohydrates, like little sponges, going to my thighs, belly, and hips.

Proponents of the Atkins Diet have scared me into believing that carbohydrates make me fat and that protein is king. Conversely, the misnomer "fat" has convinced me that even beneficial fats will make me fat.

Let's get one thing straight right now: There are no bad foods; there are only bloated portion sizes. Total calories in our day are composed of three items: fat, carbohydrates, and protein. Too much of total calories get stored as, none other than (drumroll)—body fat. Let's start being sensible about our *bodies and the way we treat them. We get in such a huff about getting the correct medications, but we put little thought into the preventative, healing powers of food. God-given, from the earth, food. Eat fruits and vegetables with reckless abandon, whole grains to fill your belly, and drink calcium to protect your bones.*

And for heaven's sake, stop being afraid of carbohydrates! To paraphrase Eleanor Roosevelt's famous quotation: No carbohydrate can make you fat without your permission.

Recipes

FAJITA PASTA   Serves: 4

1 medium yellow onion, diced
2 medium red bell peppers, chopped
2 medium yellow or orange bell peppers, chopped
2 medium green bell peppers, chopped
2 tablespoons canola oil
½ cup pork tenderloins, or chicken, leftover and ready to reheat
2 tablespoons Mrs. Dash Southwest Chipotle or Extra Spicy blend
8 ounces whole-wheat pasta, cooked and drained

Directions:

1. Boil water and cook pasta while preparing other ingredients.

2. Sauté pepper and onion in canola oil.

3. Add Mrs. Dash seasoning blend.

4. Add leftover meat and heat through.

5. Drain off extra fat from pan.

6. Serve vegetables over whole-wheat pasta.

Per serving: 363 calories, 8.8 g fat, 55.7 carbohydrate, 2.7 g fiber, 15.3 g protein.

HEIRLOOM TOMATO BENEDICT   Serves: 4

4 large multi-grain sandwich thins, toasted
4 eggs, cooked over easy
1 avocado, sliced
1 pound pineapple heirloom tomato
(about 1 large tomato)

Directions:

1. Toast sandwich thins.

2. Slice tomato.

3. Build an open-faced sandwich from the bottom-up.
   - **A.** Half of a toasted thin
   - **B.** Over easy egg
   - **C.** Tomato slices
   - **D.** Avocado

4. Use the other half of the thin to eat what falls off the sandwich!

VEGETABLE SPAGHETTI SAUCE   Serves: 8

⅛ cup vegetable broth
1 medium zucchini, chopped
1 medium yellow onion, chopped
3 tablespoons garlic, minced
½ cup basil, fresh, chopped
½ cup TVP (textured vegetable protein)
1 28 oz. can tomato puree
1 6 oz. tomato paste, unsalted
1 15 oz. can tomatoes, diced, drained

Directions:

1. Warm broth on the stove and sauté onion, garlic, and zucchini.

2. Stir in remaining ingredients.

3. Simmer for 20 minutes until heated through.

TIP
Make extra and freeze for later. Thaw in the refrigerator.

And here's a grid to help you build your own healthy salads.

SATISFACTION SOLUTION SALAD GRID   **1 serving**

Salad Greens, 2 cups	Protein, 1–2 servings	Fat, 1–2 serving	Vegetables, 1 cup	Flavor, the less the better
Spinach			Artichoke hearts	Vinegars:
Cabbage, bok choy, Chinese, green	Leftover cooked meat, 1 ounce	Olive oil, 1 teaspoon	Corn	Balsamic, white and red
Boston Lettuce	Lunch meat, 1 ounce	Canola oil, 1 teaspoon	Beets	Rice vinegar
Lamb's lettuce	Beans, ½ cup	Avocado, 1 ounce	Broccoli	Apple cider vinegar
Mesclun		Nuts, 1 ounce	Carrots	Juice:
Mizuna		Nut butter, 1 ½ teaspoon	Celery	Lime juice
Arugula		Seeds, 1 tablespoon	Cucumber	Lemon juice
Oak leaf lettuce		Cheese, 1 ounce	Onion	Orange juice
Romaine lettuce			Jicama	Pineapple juice
Watercress			Mushrooms	Grapefruit juice
Bitter greens:			Bell peppers	
Swiss chard			Tomatoes	
Collard greens			Squash	
Kale			Radishes	
Mustard greens			Water chestnuts	
Turnip greens				
Dandelion				

Top 2 cups of salad greens with protein, fat, more vegetables, and low-calorie flavorings such as vinegar to make a satisfying salad.

Satisfaction Solution: Protein

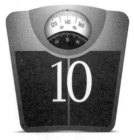

Find Out How Protein Plays a Vital Role in Weight Loss by Tamping Down Your Hunger and Helping You Feel Full on Fewer Calories

Typical American meals aren't lacking in protein (or fat) [1]. Americans love meat so much that we have meat-lovers' pizzas and the infamous Double Down Sandwich from KFC, which uses deep-fried chicken filets as its "bread."

Protein packs some power for weight loss because it helps you feel satisfied, but eating protein that's loaded with fat isn't going to get you there.

Step 1 is choosing healthy, lean animal protein and plant-based protein over their fatty cousins. Step 2 is to watch your portion sizes.

The American Institute for Cancer Research is calling it the "New American Plate": Fill your plate one-third or less with poultry, fish, or red meat. The other two-thirds should contain fruits, vegetables, whole grains, and beans. This is the optimal way to eat for weight loss and your health [2].

Protein: Why It's So Vital for Weight Loss

Protein contains amino acids, which help your body build muscle and bone. Because your body can't store amino acids, you need a daily supply of protein in your diet [1].

Protein is critical while you lose weight because it helps you maintain lean body mass while you lose fat, says Lisa Bunce [3]. It also plays a major role in how satisfied you feel. Protein takes longer than carbohydrates to break down in your stomach, making you feel full longer, Bunce says [3]. At the same time, it helps keep your blood sugar levels stable. Eating only carbohydrates (such as a plate of pasta) will cause your blood sugar levels to spike, contributing to satisfaction soon after the meal, and then drop steeply, leaving you ravenous before your next meal [3].

But protein prevents those spikes and drops in blood sugar because it stimulates the release of insulin and allows your body to use carbohydrates more effectively [4].

It's as simple as sprinkling chopped nuts on your morning oatmeal, or adding a hard-boiled egg to your salad [3].

Consider this: A large European study of 772 families found that putting adults on a diet high in protein and low on the glycemic index (which includes foods that are digested more slowly) made them less likely to quit the diet than people eating a low-protein diet that was high on the glycemic index [5].

The study begs the question: How much protein do you need? Later in this chapter you'll find a grid that tells you precisely how many grams of protein to aim for every day according to your weight. The recommendations are based on scientific evidence of what people need [4].

Your Goal: A Wide Variety of Healthy Protein

Complete protein—protein that contains all of the amino acids your body needs in one package—comes from animals, so there's good reason to include it in your diet. Incomplete protein—from plant sources—may not contain all of the essential amino acids in one specific food, but you shouldn't pass them up [1].

Eating a variety of plant proteins throughout the day will satisfy your needs for all amino acids, and while plant protein doesn't contain cholesterol and is low in fat, it's packed with fiber and will make you feel fuller longer. In addition to getting heart-healthy fiber and protein in one package, plant protein also provides phytochemicals, vitamins, and minerals [4].

> Protein plays a major role in how satisfied you feel. It takes longer to break down in your stomach, making you feel full longer.

Animal protein doesn't have fiber (although it does provide vitamins and minerals) and can be high in fat, including saturated fat that can raise blood cholesterol and put you at higher risk for heart disease and stroke [1, 6].

Sit down and eat 6 ounces of New York strip steak, and you'll get 26 grams of total fat, ten of them saturated [7]. But slide 6 ounces of baked cod onto your plate and you'll get only 1.5 grams of total fat and almost no saturated fat [8].

You can still have steak, but be sure to add in other proteins throughout the week. Whether you're eating steak, chicken, or fish, aim for a 3- or 4-ounce serving.

In the meantime, stay away from those fatty foods that can trigger binge eating—bacon is a good example—while leaving you unsatisfied. (See sidebar, *WhatWorks for Me*, on page 120.)

Plant Proteins: Get as Many as You Can

Tofu, edamame, chickpeas, lentils, beans, nuts, and seeds are wonderful sources of protein, Bunce says. They're low in fat and contain fiber to help you feel full. Lentil soups, bean salads, tofu stir-fry, steamed edamame, and nuts are all fabulous as meals and snacks [3].

For snacks, look for 100-calorie packs of raw almonds or soy-based granola bars, Bunce says [3].

If you haven't tried plant protein, make a goal of eating it at least once a week. A grassroots movement across the United States has declared Meatless Monday to be a day to get rid of the meat from your plate and replace it with plant protein. Looking for more recipes than you'll find in But I'm Hungry? Check out the Physicians Committee on Responsible Medicine's website (www.PCRM.com) for tasty recipes [4].

In a large study, researchers followed 85,168 women and 44,548 men for at least two decades. They found that those who ate a low-carb diet with plenty of plant-based proteins were healthier and had lower mortality rates, including from heart disease. Those who ate a low-carb diet high in animal protein had higher rates of death due to cancer, heart disease, and other causes [9].

While high-protein diets like Atkins, in which you eat the burger and ditch the bread, may have shed light on the power of protein for weight loss, those diets aren't sustainable, and some argue they may be bad for your health. Plant protein, on the other hand, gives you a two-in-one deal: fiber and protein. When it comes to preventing diseases such as diabetes and cancer, plant protein is the way to go, thanks to their vitamins, minerals, and phytochemicals [4].

There's been concern about soy's effect on health, particularly that it could affect the thyroid. Studies have found that soy protein (including soy milk, tofu, tempeh, miso, soy meat substitutes, and soy cheese substitutes) don't cause hypothyroidism, although soy isoflavones may affect the amount of iodine your body has to make thyroid hormone, and you may need to get more iodine if you're eating soy. Soy may also help improve cholesterol levels, lower one's risk of hip fractures related to osteoporosis, and lower one's risk of breast cancer [18].

Even better news: Plant protein benefits not only your health but also your wallet and the environment. Pound for pound, plant protein is cheaper than animal protein. (Not to mention that it carries fewer calories.) [4]

Fish and Seafood: Two to Three Times a Week

Fish and seafood are the little darlings of the protein world, Bunce says. They contain omega-3 fatty acids that keep your heart healthy. However, keep in mind that portion control is still key because too much of even a good fat is bad for your overall health. Also, beware of mercury levels. The fish with the highest levels of mercury are mackerel king, shark, swordfish, and tilefish from the Gulf of Mexico [11].

Mercury levels depend on the type of fish and where it's from. Among the best seafood choices from farms in the United States include cobia, tilapia, and freshwater salmon farmed in tank systems. The best sources of seafood that come from the Pacific Ocean include halibut and cod (from the United States, not imported). Striped bass (farmed and caught in the wild), mahi mahi from the U.S. Atlantic, and farmed arctic char are also among the best choices. For a complete and updated list of the best seafood choices and those to avoid, go to www.seafoodwatch.org [4].

What Works for Me

Ryan Sullivan, a marketing director for a home health care agency who writes the blog, No More Bacon, from Orem, UT

I call bacon a "gateway meat" because it's my trigger food. My weight-loss and healthy-living goals spiral into the gutter when I eat it. It's salty and fatty and I can't stop eating everything once it passes my lips.

For me, weight loss has been about getting rid of things like bacon and focusing on healthier foods, such as lean protein and fruits and vegetables, which I barely ate before losing weight. Instead of fatty meats, right now my protein is more likely to come from healthier sources, such as lean beef, chicken, fish, eggs, beans, nuts, and dairy.

Eating this way doesn't make me hungry, because I avoid the foods that trigger binges, and I get enough protein and a wide variety of nutrients that keep me feeling full.

When I decided to start losing weight in July 2009, I was almost four hundred pounds. Since then I've lost more than 140 pounds. At my heaviest, I was frustrated that I didn't feel well. I also saw my two little boys growing up (my youngest was around nine months old and my oldest was three years old), and I feared that I wouldn't be part of their lives.

The idea of not eating more bacon started as a joke, but the more I wrote my blog and lived the lifestyle, the more I realized that no more bacon was a real philosophy for me. I knew I would have to make sacrifices. I had to add or take away things from my everyday life in order to be healthy.

I made the lifestyle change overnight, which isn't something I'd necessarily recommend. I went to bed one night a fast-food junkie and woke up the next day swearing off bacon, fast food, and diet soda. But at the same time I added healthy foods that filled me up.

Today I feel so much better. I'm lighter and healthier; I don't feel as stressed, and our family is much more active. I don't fear that I'll miss out on my kids' lives because now I know nothing can stop me from being there.

Bunce recommends choosing salmon (which is high in omega-3s) once a week and sardines, herring, canned salmon, or smoked trout once a week. Then, add a white fish, such as cod. If you like canned tuna, limit it to 6 ounces a week. Also, don't make the mistake of thinking fish is only for dinner. Add smoked salmon to your egg whites in the morning or shrimp to your salad at lunch [3].

Lean Beef: Twice a Week

If you like red meat, go ahead and have it a couple of times a week. It's an excellent source of iron and zinc, Bunce says. Go for lean cuts of beef, such as round, sirloin, or filet mignon. And if you can find it, choose grass-fed beef because it's lower in saturated fat, Bunce says [3].

Beef jerky that is low fat, relatively low in sodium, and high in protein, is also a great snack, Bunce says [3]. However, beef jerky may contain sodium nitrate, a preservative that can make people sick. Nitrates have also been found to cause cancer in lab animals [12]. You can find nitrate-free beef jerky online at www.AmericanGrassFedBeef.com [13].

Chicken and Turkey: As Often as You Like

Chicken and turkey are great sources of lean protein, but your preparation method is key. Grill or bake it with herbs for flavor. White meat has less fat than dark meat and is the better choice, but enjoying your meals is important to feeling satisfied psychologically, so having small amounts of dark meat is okay, Bunce says [3].

Pork: Up to a Couple of Times a Week

As with beef, take care to choose lean pork cuts, such as pork tenderloin or lean pork chops. If you buy pork sausage in links that are about 1.5 ounces each, it's a great way to have built-in portion control. Also, turkey or chicken sausage is lower in fat and calories [3]. Three ounces of Italian pork sausage have 18 total grams of fat (6.4 of them saturated) and 230 calories [14]. But

3 ounces of turkey sausage contains 10.4 grams of fat (2.3 of them saturated) and 196 calories [15].

Eggs: Stick with One a Day

Eggs are a complete protein, but their yolks are high in cholesterol. The American Heart Association recommends getting no more than 300 milligrams of cholesterol a day. Since one egg yolk contains 213 milligrams, use only one egg yolk [16]. However, the whites are a great source of lean protein, so if you want more than one egg, use the egg whites [4].

Dairy: Two to Three Servings a Day

Some research has found that dairy can help people lose weight, but not all studies have been conclusive. In one study of 126 people who were followed for two years, those who got more calcium from dairy products and had higher levels of vitamin D lost more weight [17].

The takeaway is that you need calcium to keep your metabolism running, but it doesn't necessarily have to be from dairy [4]. The recommended dietary allowances for calcium are 1,000 milligrams for adult women up to age fifty and 1,200 for women after age fifty. For men, it's recommended that they get 1,000 milligrams up to age seventy and then increase it to 1,200 milligrams after age seventy [18].

Calcium is found in dairy and other sources, such as tofu, spinach, broccoli, kale, and turnip greens [18]. Your best strategy is to get calcium from dairy and nondairy sources because animal sources of dairy can cause your blood to become more acidic, which can lead to the breakdown of bones [4]. When you choose dairy, go for nonfat milk and low-fat cheese and yogurt [3].

Good-Bye, Double Down

Now you know: Protein doesn't have to come loaded with fat and calories. It's an essential part of your weight-loss plan and can help make you successful as long as you choose the right sources and stick with proper portion sizes of 3 or 4 ounces.

Scale Won't Budge? Count Your Protein Grams

Planning well-balanced meals will probably naturally give you the right amount of protein to feel satisfied. But when weight loss becomes a struggle and you're feeling unsatisfied, it may be worthwhile to start counting the number of grams of protein you're eating, says Bunce.

> When weight loss becomes a struggle and you're feeling unsatisfied, it may be worthwhile to start counting the number of grams of protein you're eating.

When her clients complain about being hungry or reach a weight-loss plateau, she looks at their protein intake. Once they start eating more protein, many start to see progress, she says [3].

The Institute of Medicine recommends aiming for at least 0.8 gram of protein for every kilogram of body weight [19]. A good rule of thumb is to get between 0.8 and 1 gram of protein per kilogram of body weight. This totals roughly 15 percent of your total daily calorie needs. Here's how it breaks down.

Weight in Pounds	Number of Grams of Protein to Aim for Every Day
150	54–68
160	58–73
170	62–77
180	66–82
190	69–86
200	73–91
215	78–98
230	83–105

Dietitian's Diary

It's Easier than You Think to Get Plant-Based Protein

Animal protein is a complete protein because in one package (meat) it contains all of the amino acids our bodies need. Plant proteins, on their own, are not complete proteins. Different plants and grains contain some, but not all, amino acids. Thus, for years vegetarians and dietitians alike thought that each meal needed to include a combination of plants, legumes/beans, and grains to make a complete protein.

What a lot of work and planning!

Thankfully, the world of nutrition research is ever evolving. We've realized that being vegetarian is much easier than we thought. The latest news is that if we eat a variety of plant proteins throughout the day we will get all the amino acids our body needs for metabolism. By introducing more plant proteins into your diet, you can not only avoid all the cholesterol and saturated fat that you get from animal protein, but you also get vitamins, minerals, phytochemicals, and fiber. When considering your waistline, health, and pocketbook, pound for pound plant protein is a better value than animal protein.

Recipes

SATISFACTION SUCCOTASH   Serves: 8

2 cups corn kernels, frozen
2 cups soybeans, frozen
2 medium tomatoes, chopped
1 orange bell pepper
½ cup red onion, diced
3 tablespoons parsley pesto

Directions:

1. Rinse soybeans and corn with room temperature water to slightly thaw.

2. Combine with remaining ingredients.

3. Serve chilled.

Per serving: 298 calories, 12.3 g fat, 27.7 g carbohydrate, 3 g fiber, 19 g protein.

ITALIAN CRUSTED SALMON WITH PESTO   Serves: 2

2 four-oz. cuts of fresh salmon
⅓ cup unbleached all-purpose flour
⅓ cup cornmeal
1 tablespoon Mrs. Dash Garlic and Herb Blend
1 tablespoon Mrs. Dash Onion and Herb Blend
2 egg whites
2 tablespoons water
2 tablespoons olive oil

Directions:

1. Mix flour through herb blends in a shallow bowl.

2. Whip together whites and water in a shallow bowl.

3. Coat salmon with egg mixture.

4. Dredge salmon in flour blend.

5. Repeat with second cut of salmon.

6. Heat one tablespoon of oil in pan on medium-low heat.

7. Cook one piece of salmon at a time.

8. Cook on one side about 5 minutes until lightly brown.

9. Flip salmon and cook another 5 minutes.

10. Repeat with second cut of salmon.

11. Top each cut with 1 tbsp of Walnut Pesto.

Without Pesto, Per serving: 239 calories, 8.2 g fat, 17.7 g carbohydrate, .1 g fiber, 23.5 g protein.

WALNUT PESTO

2 cups fresh basil, lightly packed
½ cup walnuts
1 tablespoon garlic, minced
¼ cup olive oil
3 tablespoons parmesan cheese

Directions:

1. Combine basil, walnuts, and garlic in food processor.

2. Blend for 10 seconds.

3. Continue blending while slowly adding in oil.

4. Last, blend in cheese.

Per serving: 173 calories, 16 g fat, 4.1 g carbohydrate, 1.6 g fiber, 3 g protein.

CHICKEN AND ROOT VEGETABLES (CROCK POT MEAL)   Serves: 8

4–6 lb. roasting chicken
2 leeks, sliced and washed
½ red onion, sliced
3 beets with greens
1 turnip, sliced
2 potatoes, sliced

1 tablespoon thyme
1 tablespoon oregano
1 cup water
1 teaspoon salt
½ tablespoon pepper
Canola oil cooking spray

Directions:

1. Remove beet greens and set aside.

2. Slice potatoes, onion, turnip, and beets about the same size and thickness; ¼-inch thick is best. Also, beets will turn your hands a deep pink/red. Wearing disposable kitchen gloves is recommended.

3. Mix leeks through water in crock pot.

4. Place roasting chicken atop vegetables and spray lightly to coat with oil.

5. Sprinkle salt and pepper evenly on chicken.

6. Cover chicken, like a blanket, with beet greens to seal in moisture. Greens are edible when cooking is complete!

7. Cook on high for 4 to 5 hours.

Per serving: 487 calories, 22.6 g fat, 27 g carbohydrate, 2 g fiber, 43.8 g protein.

Choosing the Right Protein Source

Use these charts to choose the right protein sources for your meals and snacks during the day. Besides calories, we've included the amount of protein, fat, and fiber each choice will give you.

Unless otherwise stated, nutrition facts are based on 3 oz. animal protein, ½ cup plant protein (beans and grains, cooked), 1 oz. cheese, ¼ cup nuts/seeds, and 8 oz.1 cup milk. Meat is broiled, roasted, or cooked using dry heat (healthiest preparation possible). The nuts and seeds are without salt. Plant proteins are prepared with water and no salt.

Meat, Fish, Legumes, and Grains

Protein Item	Calories	Protein (grams)	Fat (grams)	Fiber (grams)
Adzuki beans	147	8.5	0.1	8.5
Amaranth	125	4.6	2	3
Arctic char (farmed)	158	15.75	9.75	0
Barley	97	1.7	0.35	3
Beef tenderloin	275	20	21	0
Bison	152	22	7	0
Black beans	114	8	0.5	7.5
Black-eyed peas	90	6	1	4
Buckwheat groats	77	2.8	0.5	2
Bulgur	76	3	0.2	4.1
Cannellini (white kidney) beans	110	8	0	6
Chicken breast	142	27	3	0
Chicken leg (1 leg)	181	26	8	0
Cod	89	19.4	0.8	0
Cod (Pacific Ocean)	72	16	0.4	0
Corn	78	2.5	0.6	2
Cranberry beans	120	8	0.4	9
Eggs (1 egg white)	17	3.5	0	0
Eggs (1 hard boiled)	78	6	5	0
Farro	100	4	1	4

(Continued)

Protein Item	Calories	Protein (grams)	Fat (grams)	Fiber (grams)
Flank steak (braised)	224	23	14	0
Garbanzo beans	134	7	2	6
Great Northern beans	104	7	0.4	6
Ground beef, 95% lean	164	25	6	0
Ground beef, 90% lean	196	24	10	0
Ground beef, 85% lean	218	24	13	0
Ground chicken	161	20	9	0
Ground turkey, 85% lean	219	21	15	0
Ground turkey, 93% lean	181	23	10	0
Halibut (Pacific Ocean)	94	19	1	0
Herring	173	19.6	9.9	0
Kamut	126	5.55	0.78	3
Lamb chop/ roast	200	22	12	0
Lentils	115	8.9	0.38	8
Lima beans	108	7	0.3	6.5
Mahi mahi (U.S. Atlantic)	90	20	1	0
Millet	104	3	0.87	1
Mung beans	106	7	0.4	7.5
Navy beans	127	7.5	0.5	9.5

Protein Item	Calories	Protein (grams)	Fat (grams)	Fiber (grams)
Oats, instant	80	2.7	1.6	2
Oats, regular	303	13	5	8
Pink/calico beans	126	7.6	0.4	4.5
Pinto beans	122	7.5	0.5	7.5
Popcorn, air popped	31	1	0.36	1
Popcorn, microwave, with oil	32	0.4	2.4	0.4
Pork tenderloin	171	25	7	0
Quinoa	111	4	1.78	3
Red kidney beans	112	7.5	0.4	6.5
Rice, brown	108	2.5	0.88	2
Rice, white	103	2.1	0.2	0.3
Rice, wild	83	3.2	0.28	1.5
Rye bread (1 slice)	83	2.7	1	12
Salmon (canned)	118	17	5	0
Salmon (wild caught)	155	22	7	0
Sardines (3 fish)	75	4	4	0
Shrimp	101	19	1.5	0
Smoked trout	137	18.2	6.8	0
Sorghum	325	10.8	3.1	6
Soybeans, green	127	11	6	4
Spelt	123	5.3	0.8	4
Split peas	116	8.1	0.38	8

(Continued)

Protein Item	Calories	Protein (grams)	Fat (grams)	Fiber (grams)
Striped bass (farmed and wild caught)	105	19	2.5	0
Teff	127	4.8	0.8	3.5
Tempeh (½ cup)	160	15	9	4
Tofu (½ cup)	94	10	6	0.4
Top sirloin	207	23	12	0
Tuna (canned, in water)	99	22	1	0
Turkey breast/filet	115	26	1	0
Wheat berries	300	12	1	12

Source: USDA National Nutrient Database for Standard Reference.

Cheese

Protein Item	Calories	Protein (grams)	Fat (grams)	Fiber (grams)
American Cheese, low fat	38	5	1.4	0
Cheddar cheese	114	7	9	0
Cheddar cheese, low fat	49	7	2	0
Mozzarella cheese, part skim	72	7	4.5	0
Mozzarella cheese, whole milk	85	6	6	0
Soy cheese, 3-cheese blend (1 oz)	70	2	4	1

Protein Item	Calories	Protein (grams)	Fat (grams)	Fiber (grams)
Soy cheese, American (1 slice)	70	2	5	0
Soy cheese, Cheddar (1 oz)	63	7	3	1
Soy cheese, cheddar (1 slice)	45	3	2	0
Soy cheese, mozzarella (1 oz)	70	3	4	1
Soy cheese, mozzarella (1 slice)	70	2	5	0
Swiss cheese	108	8	8	0
Swiss cheese, low fat	48	8	1.4	0

Nuts and Seeds

Protein Item	Calories	Protein (grams)	Fat (grams)	Fiber (grams)
Almonds (¼ cup)	132	2	11	3
Brazil nuts	218	5	22	2.5
Cashews	197	5	16	1
Chestnuts	88	1	0.8	2
Flaxseed meal (2 tablespoon)	80	3	4.5	4
Hazelnuts	181	4	17	3
Macadamias	237	3	25	3
Pecans	188	2.5	20	3

(Continued)

Protein Item	Calories	Protein (grams)	Fat (grams)	Fiber (grams)
Pine nuts	227	5	23	1
Pistachios	174	6	14	3
Pumpkin seeds	71	3	3	3
Sesame seeds	206	6	18	4
Sunflower seeds	67	2.5	6	1
Walnuts	191	4.5	19	2

Satisfaction Solution: Fat

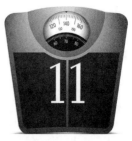

Learn About the Role Fat Plays in Weight Loss and How to Choose Healthy Fats

Major Diet Mistake: Cutting Out Too Much Fat

It's tempting to think that cutting as much fat as possible from your diet will be the key to losing weight, but it's actually the wrong thing to do.

The reality is that healthy fat is almost as important as protein at keeping you satisfied—and getting the right amount of healthy fat is part of the solution to losing weight while staying satisfied [1].

One study compared low-fat diets with diets high in protein that included a moderate amount of fat and a low-to-moderate amount of carbohydrates. Researchers found that people who ate the high-protein diet (along with more fat) lost more weight compared to those on a low-fat diet [2].

But when people decide to lose weight, it's common to see them stock up on fat-free salad dressings or low-fat cheeses, says Jessica Levinson [1].

That might not necessarily be the way to go. For one thing, fat in your diet helps your body absorb fat-soluble vitamins, such as vitamins A, D, E, and K, Levinson says. Fat in your salad dressing, for instance, helps your body absorb nutrients in the vegetables you're eating [1].

And fat also helps you feel satiated, which is your ultimate goal when you're working on losing weight without feeling hungry [1]. After all, the fat in foods is often what gives us the most pleasure.

The key phrase is *healthy fat*. We're not saying to slather your bread with gobs of butter or pour high-fat bleu cheese dressing on your salad, but a homemade salad dressing made with a tablespoon of heart-healthy olive oil— now that's a good idea! This chapter tells you what are considered healthy fats and how much you should get.

179

Healthy, Filling Fats

Together with protein and carbohydrates, dietary fat is one of the three macronutrients that give your body energy [3]. It's not something you should take out of your diet altogether, especially when healthy fats have so many health benefits, particularly for your heart.

But it's also important not to overdo it. Not only is fat packed with calories, which can ultimately lead to weight gain when you get too much, but a high-fat diet may also trigger cravings. One study of mice found that being a regular connoisseur of fatty foods may rewire the pleasure center of your brain to make you crave those foods even more. When the researchers fed mice a high-fat diet for longer than six months, their brain chemistry changed in a way to promote cravings [4].

When you're making your meals, reach for the following types of fat.

Monounsaturated Fat

Monounsaturated fats can help improve cholesterol levels and lower risk for heart disease when you eat them instead of saturated and trans fats. Studies have also found that they may even help to control blood sugar and insulin levels [3, 5].

Where to Find It

- Olive oil
- Peanut oil
- Canola oil
- Avocado oil
- Nuts and seeds
- Poultry [3]

What to Aim For

Your total fat for the day should be about 20 to 35 percent of your calories. If you're eating 1,500 calories per day, you should get 33 to 58 grams of total fat [3].

Polyunsaturated Fat

Polyunsaturated fats are found in plant-based foods and oils and may help improve cholesterol levels and offer protection from heart disease and type 2 diabetes. This type of fat includes omega-3 fatty acids, found in fish, which help lower blood pressure and protect against an irregular heartbeat [3].

Where to Find It

- Vegetable oils (such as safflower, corn, sunflower, soy, and cottonseed)
- Nut oils (such as peanut)
- Poultry
- Nuts and seeds
- Fatty, cold-water fish (such as salmon, mackerel, and herring)
- Flaxseed (which needs to be ground in order for your body to absorb it) and flax oil
- Walnuts [3]

What to Aim for

You should aim to get 20 to 35 percent of your calories from total fat, so try to get as many as you can from polyunsaturated and monounsaturated fats [3].

How do you add these healthy fats to your diet? Sprinkle slivered nuts or sunflower seeds on salads or spread nonhydrogenated peanut or other nut butters onto celery, whole-grain toast or crackers, or apple slices. Make your own salad dressing and marinade with olive oil. Use canola oil when you're baking. And put omega-3-rich fish and flaxseed on the menu twice a week [3].

The Fats to Be Wary Of

It would be unrealistic to say you should never have butter on your mashed potatoes or that you can't sink your teeth into a juicy rib ever again. But it's important to remember that unhealthy fats can do a number on your cardiovascular system. And keep in mind the potential for cravings. Odds are that when you crave food that's high in fat, it's probably something that comes from the deep fryer [4].

Saturated Fat

Too much saturated fat, which mainly comes from animal sources such as meat and whole milk, can raise your total cholesterol and your low-density lipoprotein (LDL) (bad) cholesterol levels, which in turn can increase your risk of cardiovascular disease. Saturated fat may also elevate your risk for type 2 diabetes [3].

Where to Find It

- Lard and butter
- Whole and 2% milk
- Cream
- Coconut, palm, and other tropical oils
- Cocoa butter
- Cheese and dairy products made from whole and 2% milk
- Beef, beef fat
- Veal
- Lamb
- Pork and bacon
- Poultry fat
- Sausage and hot dogs [3, 5]

What to Limit It To

Aim to get no more than 10 percent of your calories from saturated fat, but if you want to treat your heart really well, keep it below 7 percent. If you're eating 1,500 calories a day, that means getting 17 grams of your total daily grams of fat (12 if you're aiming for 7 percent). And remember that this counts toward your total fat per day and has to be added to the healthy fats in your diet [3].

Trans Fat

Although a small amount of trans fats are found in foods such as beef, pork, lamb, and butterfat, most of the trans fats we eat are processed. Food manufacturers create trans fats by hydrogenating them, which means they add hydrogen to the food because it cooks more easily and tends not to spoil. (If the serving size contains less than 0.5 gram of trans fat the processor is not legally required to list it on the label. So check the ingredients label for "partially hydrogenated-ANY oil," which translates to trans fat.) Studies show that trans fats in processed foods can raise LDL (bad) cholesterol levels and lower high-density lipoprotein (good) cholesterol levels, which puts you at risk for cardiovascular disease [3, 5].

Where to Find It

- Margarines
- Snack foods such as donuts, cookies, muffins, pies, and cakes

- French fries and other deep-fried foods
- Meat
- Dairy products [3, 5]

What to Limit It To

Ideally, we do not want to eat any trans fats. Otherwise, try to get only 1 percent of your total calories from trans fats, recommends the American Heart Association, which is less than 2 grams a day when you're eating 1,500 calories [3, 5].

What About Cholesterol?

The American Heart Association also recommends getting less than 300 milligrams a day of cholesterol, which is found in eggs, chicken, beef, hamburgers, seafood, dairy products, lard, and butter. If you have heart disease, or if your LDL cholesterol is 100 mg/dL or greater, aim to get less than 200 milligrams of cholesterol every day [5].

A large egg has 212 milligrams of cholesterol, so paying attention to the amount of cholesterol listed on food labels is a good idea [6].

Healthy Fats: Using a Light Hand

Even when you're cooking with healthy fats, it's important to use them sparingly; when a tablespoon of olive oil packs in 120 calories, a little bit goes a long way.

Here are some ways to use a light hand when you're preparing meals with healthy fats.

- Use a measuring spoon when you're adding oil to a pan for cooking or when making homemade salad dressing, rather than pouring it from the bottle and losing sight of how much you're getting, Levinson suggests [1].
- Almost any vegetable (from potatoes and yams to carrots, mushrooms, squash, and cauliflower) tastes wonderful when coated with oil and roasted in the oven. But rather than drizzling the oil onto the vegetables, measure the oil and pour it into a little bowl and then brush it onto the vegetables before roasting [1].
- Skip fat-free salad dressings and go for the full-fat or reduced-fat versions, but be sure to measure how much you're using. Levinson recommends sticking with one tablespoon of full-fat dressing or two tablespoons of reduced-fat dressing [1].

- Keep in mind that two tablespoons of peanut butter will give you 188 calories. Just as you would for oils and salad dressings, measure out the nut butters with a measuring spoon before you spread it on your bread or fruit [7].

- Add just a few shavings or crumbles of flavorful cheese to your meal to give it lots of flavor without too much fat. Some good choices: fresh parmesan, Pecorino Romano, Gruyère, feta, goat cheese, bleu cheese, cheddar, or Gouda.

Weight loss doesn't have to mean depriving yourself of the good stuff. It means making an effort to get fat from the healthiest sources you can and being careful about how much you use.

What Works for Me

Heidi Mitchell, a customer service representative who lives in Milwaukie, OR

Up until a year and a half ago, I had been in denial about my weight and the high-fat diet I was eating every day. After years of yo-yo dieting, I had given up. When I looked in the mirror, I thought to myself, "I'm not really that fat."

Then my friend and I vowed to start Weight Watchers together. I thought my weight was in the two-hundreds because I had always told myself I would never get over three hundred. That day at Weight Watchers I stepped on the scale, and it said 312.

I cried, but then I got myself together, and I started learning how to eat the right way. At the time, I worked an overnight shift, from midnight to 8 a.m. When I was home during the day, I wanted to spend as much time with my husband and kids as I could, so I hadn't been taking the time to make myself a dinner to eat at work. Instead, I used my twenty-five-minute break to drive to a fast-food restaurant, order the biggest meal I could, scarf it down and head back to work.

That's one of the first things I changed. I went to the supermarket and bought all of my favorite fruits and vegetables: strawberries, blackberries, raspberries, bananas, oranges, cantaloupe, watermelon, cauliflower, broccoli, brussels sprouts, spinach, and jicama. Then I bought Ziploc steamer bags.

Instead of getting greasy drive-thru meals, I started steaming meat, fish, and vegetables in the microwave to eat at home and at work. And jicama became my new snack. I love slicing it and eating it raw. I had been salting everything I ate, but I started using oregano, basil, and garlic to flavor my food.

I was also trying lots of new recipes, such as chicken with applesauce and cinnamon. At the same time, I got junk food out of the house. After eighteen months I had lost 102 pounds.

Thankfully, I work a different shift now—5 a.m. to 1 p.m.—so my sleep schedule is a little easier, although some nights I still go to bed too late.

One thing that really helps: physical activity. If I've had a strenuous day at work, my instinct is to come home, sit on the couch or at the computer and veg for the rest of the day. But when I push myself to get out and take an hour-long walk I feel better for the rest of the day, and I sleep better at night. On my days off I put on a weighted vest and go for a five-mile hike, and I love it.

I stay motivated by connecting with others online. I have a Heidi's Weight-Loss Page on Facebook, and I track my workouts and share them with friends online at SportyPal.com.

After all this time I still have cravings to go back to my old habits. A couple of months ago I had a craving for a Jack In the Box bacon and egg biscuit. (I used to have two of those every morning). But instead of heading straight to the restaurant, I went online to find out how many points it would cost me. It was about twelve—almost half of the thirty points I eat a day. That clinched it: I'd rather stick to my plan.

I notice that stress still triggers unhealthy eating, and it's something I'm working on. In the meantime, my husband has been a great support. I'm feeling so good about the progress I've made that I signed up to do a half-marathon in 2012 at Walt Disney World.

Smart, Low-Fat Switches

Nutritionists don't recommend snacking on a lot of low-fat or fat-free products like crackers and cookies because they often have added sugar, and they're not going to make you feel satisfied the way whole foods will.

However, there are times when choosing a low-fat alternative is a smart thing to do. Here are some low-fat recommendations.

One note about cheeses: Some nutritionists recommend using the full-fat versions of high-flavor cheeses, such as parmesan or cheddar. Because they have so much flavor you'll only need a small amount in your food, but you'll get the satisfying taste.

Here's a guide to help you choose low-fat alternatives [8, 5].

Instead of ...	Try ...
Oil, shortening, butter, or lard	Nonstick cooking spray
Regular margarine	Soft margarine labeled "0 grams trans fat"

(Continued)

Instead of ...	Try ...
Whole milk	Low-fat (1%) or fat-free milk
Regular mayonnaise	Avocado mayonnaise made with olive or canola oil or reduced-fat mayonnaise. One good example is Vegenaise, from Follow Your Heart products.
Ice cream	Low-fat or fat-free frozen yogurt or ice cream, sherbet, or sorbet
Sour cream	Plain low-fat yogurt or tangy Greek yogurt
Cream cheese	Neufchatel (low-fat) or light cream cheese
Whole-milk mozzarella or ricotta cheese	Part-skim milk mozzarella or ricotta cheese, or crumbled frozen tofu
Whipping cream	Imitation whipped cream made with fat-free milk
American, cheddar, Swiss, jack, and cottage cheeses	Reduced-calorie, low-calorie, reduced-fat, low-fat, or fat-free cheeses
Coffee cream (half and half) or nondairy powder or liquid creamer	1% or 2% milk or fat-free dry milk powder or soy milk, which has the thicker consistency of cream
Granola	Reduced-fat granola, oatmeal, cooked grits, bran flakes, or other lower fat, high-fiber cereals with lots of fruits and nuts
Pasta alfredo or with another cheese sauce	Pasta marinara or pasta primavera
Ramen noodles	Rice or a healthier noodle, such as whole-wheat spaghetti or macaroni
Regular ground beef	Extra-lean ground beef, such as ground round, or ground turkey or vegetarian meat substitutes. One company that produces a whole line of meat substitutes is Quorn Foods.
Chicken or turkey with the skin	White meat chicken or turkey without the skin
Pork, such as spareribs or un-trimmed loin	Pork tenderloin or trimmed, lean smoked ham
Bacon or sausage	Canadian bacon, lean ham, turkey, chicken, or vegetarian sausage

Instead of ...	Try ...
Regular lunch meat	Low-fat lunch meat
Breaded or fried fish	Unbreaded fish or shellfish that's not fried
French fries	Homemade or store-bought baked fries
Whole eggs	Egg whites or egg substitutes
Cream soups	Broth-based soups
High-fat frozen dinners	Frozen dinners with less than 13 grams of fat per serving (preferably low in sodium)
Pound, chocolate, or yellow cake	Angel food cake

 ## Dietitian's Diary

Butter vs. Margarine

The debate has raged for years. Butter or margarine: Which is the lesser of the two evils? They both have their cardiovascular downfalls. One of the biggest differences is that butter is created by a simple process (churning), while margarine is created through the chemical process of hydrogenation. Sure, the amounts of calories also differ between the two. The type and amount of fat in both products vary as well. When comparing the two, however, you cannot simply look at calories. The main issues of the debate on butter vs. margarine stem from the type of fats that compose them.

Butter

Butter is essentially the fat of the milk. It is created by churning whole milk into a delicious yellow spread. The flavor creates the standard for all imitation spreads thereafter. The fat that composes butter is mostly saturated fat. In a 1-tablespoon serving of butter there are approximately 11 grams of fat. Seven of those 11 grams are saturated fat. There are also omega unsaturated fats in the total unsaturated fat of butter (3.5 g/unsaturated fat). One of the upsides to butter, in comparison to margarine, is that it has no trans fats, which have been found to negatively affect your body's cholesterol faster than saturated fats. You can also get real organic butter made from certified organic milk. If butter is your choice of taste in moderation, try Organic Valley Products (http://www.organicvalley.coop/).

Margarine

There are several types of margarine. It can be purchased in liquid, soft (tub), or hard (stick) forms. The oil that it is made from can be anything from cottonseed to olive oil. There is also yogurt-based margarine on the market. Regardless of the origination of the fat source, all margarine is created by heating liquid oil along with a metal catalyst and hydrogen [9]. This process, called hydrogenation, creates trans fats. Legally, if there is less than 0.5 gram of trans fats per serving, the manufacturer can print "zero grams of trans fats" on the nutrition label and advertise it as being "trans-fat-free" (with an asterisk reminding you this is per serving). Be sure to look for the ingredients, and if you see partially hydrogenated oil (any type of oil) there are trans fats in the product.

The result of the hydrogenation of oil is a white, semisolid substance. The less hydrogenated the oil, the softer the resulting margarine (the liquid form, most commonly found as spray margarine, being the least hydrogenated). Once flavoring, salt, preservatives, and yellow coloring are added, it looks and tastes like butter. Margarine has the delightful flavor and color of butter with fewer calories. An average margarine (vegetable oil based) has 8 grams of fat in a tablespoon. Of those 8 grams, 2 grams are saturated and 1 gram is trans fats.

My verdict: It's up to you! Yes, it would be easier if I just gave you a straight answer, but the only real advice I can give is to practice moderation in using both. You are basically choosing between trans fats (margarine) and saturated fat (butter). Choose wisely, and follow your heart.

Recipes

TROPICAL TOFU SMOOTHIE   Serves: 2

½ cup tofu, silken
½ cup orange juice
½ cup soy milk, light, plain
1 cup pineapple chunks, canned, no juice
1 banana
4 tablespoons flaxseed meal

Directions:

1. Combine all in blender or food processor.
2. Blend until smooth.
3. Add more liquid to desired consistency.

Per serving: 276 calories, 6.4 g fat, 44.9 g carbohydrate, 3 g fiber, 9.6 g protein.

SMOKY SWEET CORN RISOTTO   **Serves: 8**

6 cups vegetable broth
¼ cup canola oil
2 cups yellow onions, chopped
1 leek, halved and sliced
2 cups short-grain brown rice (brown risotto rice)
1 cup white wine
1 15 oz. can corn, drained
1 tablespoon liquid smoke
1 teaspoon lemon zest
⅓ teaspoon pepper, ground
4 green onions, thinly sliced

Directions:

1. Keep vegetable broth warm on the stove.
2. In a nonstick pot, heat canola oil and sauté onion and leeks until translucent.
3. Add rice and toss to coat with mixture. Continuously move rice until it lightens.
4. Add white wine and simmer for about 2 minutes, continuously stirring.
5. Add one ladle of vegetable broth at a time.
6. Continuously stir until most of the broth is absorbed.
7. Continue this over the next 30 minutes until rice is soft to the taste.
8. When rice is done, stir in corn, zest, liquid smoke, and pepper and heat through.
9. Top with onions to serve.

Per serving: 348 calories, 10.2 g fat, 59.3 g carbohydrate, 3.8 g fiber, 4.8 g protein.

CRISPY BAKED GARLIC CHICKEN STRIPS   Serves: 6

4 tablespoons olive oil, extra virgin
⅛ teaspoon chili powder
2 tablespoon Herbs de Provence
2 cups all-purpose flour
1 cup nonfat milk
2 egg whites
3 cups panko bread crumbs
2 tablespoons garlic, minced
12 ounces chicken breast tenders, boneless, skinless
Sea salt and fresh ground pepper, to taste

Directions:

1. Preheat oven to 350 degrees F.
2. Put ingredients in three separate bowls for breading: flour with Herbs de Provence and chili powder (salt and pepper to taste), milk and egg whites, and bread crumbs with garlic.
3. Dredge chicken in flour, then the egg mix, then bread crumbs.
4. Re-dredge each tender in the egg mix and bread crumb mix. This will help make the chicken nice and crunchy.
5. Lay chicken onto a baking tray lined with parchment paper.
6. Refrigerate for about 15 minutes in order for breading to set.
7. Remove chicken from refrigerator and lightly spray with cooking spray.
8. Cook for 35 to 40 minutes at 350 degrees.

Per serving: 270 calories, 9.4 g fat, 25.7 g carbohydrate, 0.1 g fiber, 20.7 g protein.

Satisfaction Solution: Fiber

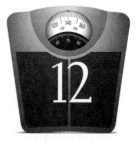

Learn How Fiber Can Make You Feel More Satisfied

An orange or a glass of orange juice? Which do you think will make you feel fuller? No surprise, it's the orange. Actually, you might even be able to drink the equivalent of four oranges before you'd feel as satisfied as you would if you just ate the fruit [1].

A big reason for that: fiber [1].

Research has found that fiber plays a huge role in satiety and weight. When researchers ask people about their diets and their body mass index, they have found that people who tend to eat a low-fiber, high-fat diet are more likely to be overweight and obese compared with people who eat high-fiber, low-fat foods [2].

It's probably why something like the apple diet has taken off in some areas of the United States. Judy Simon, RD, a clinical dietitian at the University of Washington Family Medical Center in Seattle, WA, heard about the diet from her patients. It sounds like a fad diet until you hear how it works: eat three apples a day and follow each with a healthy meal [1].

"People were losing weight," she says. "It makes sense. If you eat a higher fiber food first, you'll feel more satisfied" [1].

Research even backs it up. In a five-week study of fifty-eight adults, researchers broke them up into four groups and gave each group either nothing, an apple, applesauce, or apple juice before eating lunch. Those who ate the whole fruit ended up taking in 15 percent fewer calories at lunch compared to those who didn't have anything. (This is 300 fewer calories for a person usually eating 2,000 calories a day. That is about half a pound a week!) They also ate less than those who ate applesauce or drank juice [3].

Simon has seen the results with her own eyes. One of her patients weighed more than five hundred pounds and was planning to have weight-loss surgery, but she started eating healthier on her own before going under the knife.

One of her techniques: she decided to eat her vegetable first, then her fruit, followed by protein, and grains last, Simon says.

"In the past, she would have dug into her mashed potatoes, but if she had the veggies and fruit first when she was most hungry, that helped her feel more satisfied by the end," Simon says.

She lost 120 pounds in nine months eating that way—*before* she had the surgery.

What's the magic behind fiber? Let's find out.

So, Why Is It So Filling?

For one thing, fiber gives you the feeling of fullness in your stomach, Simon says [1]. Think about how much bulk an apple provides compared to a glass of apple juice—for fewer calories. A medium apple has just 95 calories and takes up some space in your stomach. One cup of apple juice, on the other hand, has a concentrated 120 calories and doesn't leave your stomach feeling quite so full [4].

Fiber-rich foods also take longer to eat because they require more chewing. Eat a sandwich with whole grain bread, and you'll have to work on it more than you would soft, white bread, which practically melts in your mouth. And when you take longer to eat, your brain has a chance to catch up with your stomach and register when you're full [5].

And there's another reason fiber helps you feel satisfied: It helps keep your blood sugar levels more steady, which is your goal for feeling fuller between meals. When blood sugar levels spike from eating simple sugars or refined carbs like white bread, it causes insulin to be released and a steep drop in blood sugar, which then makes you feel hungry again. But eating foods with fiber—whole-wheat bread instead of white—allows your blood sugar to rise and fall more gradually, which keeps you full longer.

You might say white sugar and refined foods are Americans' downfall because of their effect on blood sugar levels, and, unfortunately, they're ubiquitous in our diet. Fiber offers a solution. Filling up on fiber means you won't even want to indulge in unhealthy snacks between meals.

On top of that, foods that are high in fiber also tend to be full of extra nutrients, such as B vitamins and vitamin E, Simon says [1]. When your diet gives you the nutrients your body craves, you'll feel more satisfied and will be able to pass up a midnight snack more easily.

Even More Benefits

Fiber makes you feel full. What's more to love? Actually, there's plenty more to love about fiber.

It Can Protect Your Heart

Getting plenty of fiber in your diet has been associated with lower risk of heart disease in several large studies, according to Harvard School of Public Health. Studies have also found that eating fiber-rich whole grains may protect against metabolic syndrome, a group of risk factors that raise the risk of heart disease and diabetes, because it helps lower cholesterol [6].

It Can Lower Your Risk for Type 2 Diabetes

Studies have found that eating a diet rich in fiber from grains seems to lower the risk of type 2 diabetes, particularly in a diet with plenty of foods low on the glycemic index, (meaning foods that don't cause spikes in blood sugar). Meanwhile, people who eat diets with low amounts of the fiber that comes from grains but high amounts of foods high on the glycemic index (which causes your blood sugar to rise sharply) may double their risk of type 2 diabetes [6].

It Helps Prevent Inflammation of the Intestine

Diverticulitis happens to one-third of people older than forty-five and two-thirds of people older than eighty-five, but dietary fiber (especially insoluble fiber, found in barley, tomatoes, brown rice, and other high-fiber foods) may lower the risk for this painful disease, according to studies [6].

It Will Keep You Regular

Eating fiber, especially wheat bran and oat bran, can help you prevent constipation [6].

Where Can We Get Some?

Fiber is all over the place: in whole grains, vegetables, fruits, and beans. It only takes a little effort to get it into your diet, so there's really no excuse—and no reason—to skimp on this Satisfaction Solution [7].

First, find out where fiber comes from. It's the part of the plant that the body doesn't digest, so it passes through your stomach and intestines without getting broken down and absorbed. Along the way, though, it serves some good purposes [5].

The following sections describe how fiber is typically classified and what each type does.

Insoluble Fiber

This type of fiber helps keep things moving along in your digestive system, which means it can prevent constipation. Wheat bran, whole-wheat flour, nuts, and vegetables are some examples of insoluble fiber [5].

Soluble Fiber

This type of fiber dissolves in water and becomes gel-like. As it journeys through your digestive tract it helps lower your blood sugar and cholesterol. Oats, peas, beans, apples, citrus fruits, carrots, barley, and psyllium all contain soluble fiber [5].

Your goal should be to get a good mix of insoluble and soluble fiber from whole grains, fruits, vegetables, beans, peas, legumes, nuts and seeds.

Follow these rules when you're shopping in order to go high fiber.

Choose Foods Over Supplements

The foods provide vitamins and minerals that you can't get from supplements like Metamucil and Citrucel [5].

Go for Whole Foods Over Processed Foods

It's always healthier to eat the whole food rather than processed foods, but canned fruits actually retain fiber through the canning process. White bread, white pasta, and cereal that's not made from whole grain don't have as much fiber because the outer layer of the bran was stripped when it was refined [5].

Look for Unprocessed, Whole Grains

The USDA's MyPlate says to make one-quarter of your plate grains—and at least half of those grains should be whole grains. So, what do you choose? Try these, and remember that you may have to head to the whole-foods section of your supermarket or a health food store to find some of them.

- Rolled oats
- Muesli
- Whole-wheat cereal
- Oats, steel cut
- Kasha
- Millet, hulled
- Bulgur wheat
- Barley, hulled
- Buckwheat
- Brown rice
- Wild rice

- Rye
- Cornmeal (polenta)
- Wild rice
- Amaranth
- Kamut grain
- Quinoa
- Sorghum
- Spelt berries
- Wheat berries
- Popcorn
- Whole-grain barley
- Whole-grain cornmeal
- Whole-wheat bread and crackers
- Whole-wheat pasta
- Whole-wheat rolls and buns
- Whole-wheat tortillas [8, 9]

Be sure to read the directions on how to prepare the grains. Some grains, such as spelt berries and wheat berries, need to soak overnight before being cooked [9].

Buy Cereals with at Least 5 Grams of Fiber Per Serving

Such cereals often have "bran" or "fiber" in the name. If your favorite cereal doesn't qualify as high fiber, add three tablespoons of wheat bran to it, along with flaxseed meal [5].

Check the Ingredients List for Whole Grains

It's easy to buy what you think is whole-wheat bread only to find that it's refined. To be sure you're buying high-fiber bread, check the ingredients list. "Whole wheat," "whole-wheat flour," or another whole grain should be the first ingredient listed. Another good choice: breads that have at least 2 grams of fiber per serving [5].

The same goes for pita bread, cornbread, corn and flour tortillas, couscous, crackers, noodles, and pasta. Most include refined grains, but you may be able to find some that include whole grains. Look for "whole grain" or "whole wheat" on the ingredients list. For a great guide in choosing whole grains, check out the web site (http://www.wholegrainscouncil.org/) of the Whole Grains Council [8].

How Much Should You Aim For?

The National Academy of Sciences Institute of Medicine recommends that women who are fifty and younger get 25 grams of fiber a day, while older women should aim for about 21 grams a day. Men age fifty and younger should aim for 38 grams of fiber a day, while older men should try to get around 30 grams a day [5].

Here's what 38 grams of fiber looks like:

Three-quarters of a cup of bran flakes: 5 grams

Half-cup of blueberries: 2 grams

Two slices of 100 percent whole-grain bread: 4 grams

Half of an eggplant, sliced and grilled: 8 grams

Medium apple: 4.5 grams

One cup of brown rice: 3.5 grams

One cup of carrots: 3.5 grams

One cup of broccoli: 2.5 grams

Medium pear: 5 grams

If your diet doesn't have a lot of fiber in it already, be sure to increase your intake slowly over a few weeks or else you might experience gas, bloating, and cramping. As you do, drink more water because the fiber will absorb the water and help to make you regular [5]. (Check out Chapter 13 for more info on hydration.)

Sneaking in More Filling Fiber

Getting more of this nutrient can be as simple as adding high-fiber foods to the meals you already make.

Instead of juice: Eat the whole fruit. It packs more fiber for fewer calories [7].

In cereal: Fill your bowl with cereals made with kamut, kasha (which is buckwheat), or spelt, and add flaxseed meal [10].

In yogurt: Add oats with fresh fruit, such as fresh berries, sliced peaches, mango chunks, or melon.

On toast: Add slices of pear or apple with your nut butter.

In salads: Toss in tabbouleh, cooked wheat berries, or beans [10].

In sandwiches: Save the burgers for another day and grill up zucchini, onion, yellow squash, bell peppers, Portobello mushrooms, or eggplant and slap them between two slices of whole-grain bread.

In meatballs, burgers, or meatloaf: Stir in three-quarters of a cup of oats or bulgur wheat per pound of beef or turkey you use [10].

Instead of steak: Brush a big, meaty Portobello mushroom with olive oil, season with salt and pepper, and grill or sauté it.

On the grill: Throw on thick slices of pineapple or peaches lightly brushed or sprayed with oil.

In kebabs: Slide on plenty of marinated vegetables, such as onions, mushrooms, bell peppers, squash, zucchini, eggplant, or tomatoes. Or make a fruit kebab with chunks of melon, banana, pineapple, and grapes.

In spaghetti sauce: Finely chop vegetables like broccoli, mushrooms, and carrots, and add them to sauce. You can also skip the meat completely to add more fiber with more beans and vegetables, which are low/nonfat and high in fiber.

In burritos: Fold in beans and fresh salsa with lean meat and cheese.

In chilis: Add in as many beans and vegetables as you can, including corn, carrots, tomatoes, bell peppers, onions, mushrooms, zucchini, and squash. You can also add Quorn grounds or bulgur wheat.

In soups: Make a hearty vegetable soup with onion, peas, spinach, cabbage, carrots, celery, onion, mushrooms, broccoli, yams, or any other vegetables you have on hand. Also add whole-wheat pasta, barley, wheat berries, and brown or wild rice.

In salsas: Use mango or watermelon salsas as side dishes with meat.

On pizzas: Pile it with your favorite vegetables, such as mushrooms, broccoli, tomatoes, fresh spinach, bell peppers, or onions.

In bread stuffing: Add half a cup of cooked bulgur wheat, barley, or wild rice [10].

In risottos, pilafs, and other rice dishes: Use barley, brown rice, bulgur wheat, millet, quinoa, or sorghum [10].

In pasta dishes: Use whole-grain pasta or pasta that's a blend of white and whole grain [10].

In cornbread, corncakes, or corn muffins: Use whole corn meal [10].

For snacks: Grab carrot chips or other raw vegetables instead of potato chips, toasted whole-wheat pitas rather than tortilla chips, and air-popped popcorn over pretzels [6].

In cookies, muffins, breads, and pancakes: Use half whole-wheat flour and half white flour in your recipes [10].

What Works for Me

Janice Taylor is a life and weight-loss-success coach, hypnotherapist and author of the weight loss classic Our Lady of Weight Loss: Miraculous and Motivational Musings from the Patron Saint of Permanent Fat Removal (on Oprah's self-help reading list three years running!)

I most certainly did not wake one morning with a smile on my face and enthusiastically say, "Whoopee, I'm fatter than ever. I'll go on a diet. This will be fun!"

No. I rolled out of bed, pulled up my size XXL elastic-band pants and said, "Oh my, even these are tight. I must stop the fat monster from further multiplying before HE takes me over entirely." I prayed for guidance.

That's when Our Lady of Weight Loss entered the picture. "Who is Our Lady? Where did she come from?" you ask.

I often wonder! Perhaps, she is a higher power, the higher self, the good mother that lives within each of us, or maybe—as my mother likes to say—she is just a Fig Newton of my wild imagination. Does it really matter?

What matters is that instead of eating crazy amounts of fried foods, heavily buttered bread, and chocolate in any form, I was able to permanently remove more than fifty pounds of excess weight ten years ago.

Our Lady of Weight Loss taught me that I am good enough, that it's okay to love myself and believe in myself, and to focus on the outcome, not the process! Instead of setting a fifty-pound weight-loss goal, I set out to have a good time, to journey on the lighter side of weight loss and life. In other words, I lightened up in as many ways as I could! And bonus: I found my waist!

I took one small, happy, light step at a time, and permanently removed more than fifty pounds of excess weight. It's been off for ten years now—an entire decade. I have no plans to find it (again)!

I'm now a hypnotherapist and life- and weight-loss-success coach who works nationwide. I love what I do, and I am dedicated to helping any and all who want to permanently shed those extra pounds!

Remember, it's not about your weight; it's about your life! Fill up on happiness and just see what might happen!

To learn more about Janice, go to www.ourladyofweightloss.com.

Give It a Try—You'll Like It

Not only is fiber filling and nutritious, but also it tastes pretty darned good. (Don't believe the commercials that imply high-fiber foods taste like cardboard.)

But you'll enjoy fiber-rich foods more if you know what to do with them. Steamed zucchini without much seasoning may not rock your world, but turning the vegetable into a cheesy zucchini boat might.

Plus, grains like quinoa and barley will taste a little plain unless you kick them up with some flavor. Simon recommends seeking out recipes (you can start with the ones in this book) that will help you prepare high-flavor grains so you'll want to make them again and again.

Dietitian's Diary

Beans Without Fear

Beans, beans, the musical fruit. The more you eat ... You know the rest. What causes the toots anyway? Beans contain a type of carbohydrate called oligosaccharides (OS). Other types of this carbohydrate that are found in vegetables are fructo-oligosaccharides and galacto-oligosaccharides. This is not fiber. It just so happens that fiber and OS come from similar products: fruits, vegetables, and most commonly beans. FYI: Combining beans with onions, garlic, or any cabbage-family vegetable is not something to do on a first date. Dis-as-ter!

OS are carbohydrates that do not completely break down in the body. The part that our body does not absorb helps to feed the friendly bacteria in our intestines and suppress the bad bacteria. Making a long metabolic story short, friendly bacteria strengthen our immune system and produce vitamin K and biotin. Just as a human by-product of life is to breathe out carbon dioxide, the byproduct of bacteria breaking down the bean sugar creates gas in our intestines. And this gas needs out!

Let's put protein into perspective. A slice of deli meat is about 7 grams of protein. A half-cup of cooked beans is 7 grams of protein. What will you feel fuller eating? The beans. Why? Beans contain fiber. Fiber makes us feel fuller longer. There's no fiber in the meat.

By eating all these beans and vegetables does this mean you'll have a cloud of stench around you resembling Charlie Brown's friend Pig Pen? Not if you gradually increase the amount of beans in your diet. This allows the body to adjust to the amount of OS you are consuming. Other things that help with the gas: drinking plenty of water during the day and eating fruits and vegetables to help move things through and out of your colon. Also, if you cook the beans yourself (highly recommended) make sure to soak them overnight and cook in fresh water.

There are, of course, over-the counter medications to help with the gas and bloating. Or you could skip the medications and decrease the amount of beans you are eating for now. This is a process, a marathon of sorts, for our bodies. And, like a marathon, it requires patience.

Recipes

CABBAGE PASTA STEW   Serves: 12

3 tablespoons olive oil, extra virgin
3 tablespoons garlic, minced
1 medium leek, sliced and washed
1 12 oz. package brussel sprouts, frozen
4 cups savoy cabbage, chopped, about 1 head
2 cups corn, frozen, unsweetened
4 cups water
¼ cup white wine vinegar
1 medium lemon juice, fresh
1 teaspoon thyme, dried
24 ounces whole-wheat pasta, cooked

Directions:

1. Cook pasta while preparing remaining ingredients.
2. Cook frozen brussels sprouts half the amount of time as the package directions—Just enough time to soften.
3. Drain off water and cut sprouts in half.
4. In a medium- depth pan, sauté garlic and leek in olive oil.
5. Add sprouts and cabbage to pan and toss to coat with garlic mixture.
6. Add remaining ingredients (except pasta) and bring to a boil.

7. Simmer about 20 minutes or until cabbage is wilted and soft.

8. Serve in soup bowls atop cooked whole-wheat pasta (about ¼ cup pasta each).

Per serving: 305 calories, 4.5 g fat, 56 g carbohydrate, 2.9 g fiber, 10.3 g protein.

BLACK BEAN DIP   Serves: 8

1 5 oz. can black beans, drained and rinsed
1 cup salsa
3 tablespoons cilantro, fresh, chopped

Directions:

1. Combine salsa and beans in a blender or food processor.

2. Blend until smooth.

3. Stir in or top with cilantro.

Per serving: 81 calories, 0.3 g fat, 14.7 carbohydrate, 1.2 g fiber, 4.9 g protein.

WHOLE-WHEAT VEGETABLE PIZZA   Serves: 4

1 12 oz. package whole-wheat pizza dough
1 cup tomato sauce
½ cup yellow onion, diced
1 tablespoon garlic, minced
2 tablespoon olive oil, extra virgin
2 cup spinach leaves
8 ounces mozzarella cheese, low fat

Directions:

1. Cook pizza dough according to package.

2. In a stovetop pan, sauté garlic and onion until onion is translucent.

3. Stir in spinach leaves and wilt.

4. Build pizza from the bottom up:
   A. Pizza crust
   B. Sauce
   C. Spinach mixture
   D. Slices of mozzarella

5. Cook according to pizza dough package or until cheese is melted.

Per serving: 321 calories, 9 g fat, 50.5 g carbohydrate, 3.9 fiber, 9.6 g protein.

Satisfaction Solution: Water

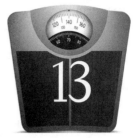

Find Out Why It's So Critical to Be Properly Hydrated

It's a mantra you've probably heard hundreds of times before: Drink plenty of water.

What's so critical about water? It assists in transporting nutrients, helps with digestion (including fiber), keeps your body a comfortable temperature, and flushes waste [1, 2]. Drinking water regularly may even lower the risk of colorectal and bladder cancers [3].

For you, right now, as you start eating healthier and watching the scale, the most important job for water will be to help you shed pounds—and it really can.

Studies have found that when people drink two glasses of water before sitting down to a meal, they eat 75 to 90 fewer calories. In one study presented at a meeting of the American Chemical Society, researchers took forty-eight people between age fifty-five and seventy-five and put them on a low-calorie diet for twelve weeks. Half drank two glasses of water three times a day before their meals, while the other half didn't. After twelve weeks, the group that drank water lost about five pounds more than those who didn't drink water [4].

There are at least two things going on: Water literally fills up your stomach and makes you feel full for no calories whatsoever. And the water was probably being swapped for high-calorie drinks like soda and juice [4]. A tall glass of water will quench your thirst just as well (if not better) as 11 ounces of lemonade, which carries 176 calories along with it [5].

But there's more to water and weight loss. Staying hydrated is key to staying in touch with true hunger signals, and research shows it may even increase your metabolism [2].

The Water and Weight-Loss Connection

Here's how water plays such a big role in weight loss.

It Can Make You Feel Less Hungry

Unfortunately, it's easy to mistake dehydration for hunger. When you feel the urge to dive into a box of crackers in the middle of the day, you might actually need a tall glass of water instead. When you're hungry, drink a glass of water and wait to see if the urge to eat goes away before you decide to have a snack [1, 2].

Be warned that when you're thirsty you might even crave salt because your body wants you to drink water, says Kate Hawley, RD, clinical dietitian at Maine Medical Center in Portland, Maine [1].

It Helps Keep Portions in Check

If you drink two cups of water before a meal, as people did in the medical studies to lose weight, a good portion of your stomach volume is being filled up with a calorie-free liquid, Hawley says. You'll have less room for food, so portion control doesn't seem so difficult [1].

It's a Great Substitute for High-Calorie Drinks

Do you really want the 177 calories in 16 ounces of sweetened iced tea when you could quench your thirst with a zero-calorie water [5]?

It Speeds up Your Metabolism

In one study of fourteen adults, researchers asked them to drink 500 milliliters of water (just under 17 ounces) and then measured their metabolism. Within ten minutes of drinking, their metabolism rose. Within thirty to forty minutes, their metabolic rate had increased by 30 percent [6].

It Gives You More Satisfaction From Your Food

Food that has a lot of water gives you volume in exchange of a smaller amount of calories, so that means you'll feel satisfied when you're finished eating. Think about the warm, full feeling you get after finishing a bowl of soup. That's what we're talking about.

First, Drink Up

The Institute of Medicine of the National Academy of Sciences advises that you let your thirst guide how much water you drink [7]. But we all know how a busy, stress-filled day can cause us to neglect the basics: food, water, bathroom breaks. Because it's easy to confuse thirst with hunger, it's probably better to aim to drink a certain number of glasses of water a day.

General recommendations for water consumption, according to the Institute of Medicine, are about 91 ounces a day for women and about 125 ounces a day for men. Those recommendations include both food and water. Typically, people get 20 percent of their water from food, so that means women should get about nine glasses of fluid a day and men should get about twelve [7].

Of those nine to twelve cups of fluid, aim for eight to ten of them to be nonalcoholic and calorie free. Keep in mind, though, that if you're in intense heat, you may need more [2].

Here are some tips on making sure you're getting enough.

Get a To-Go Cup or Bottle to Carry with You

It might help to get a cup that you designate specifically for water that will go easily from home to your car to your desk at work. The stores are stocked with so many different options for nondisposable water bottles and cups today (thanks to the eco-friendly movement that discourages using disposable water bottles to cut down on waste) that you can find them virtually everywhere [1].

If you buy one that's 16 ounces, remember that you'll need to refill it about five times a day to reach your goal of eight to ten glasses a day [2].

Sip Frequently Throughout the Day

Try to make a habit of sipping from your water cup while you work, while you drive in your car, while you're cooking, and at other times throughout the day. You don't want to get to the point where you have a dry mouth, Hawley says [1].

Always Pair a Meal with Water

About 75 percent of people's fluid intake happens while they're sitting down and eating. Rather than turning to high-calorie, sweetened drinks like juice, put water in your glass at dinner [2].

Keep Water Handy When You're Exercising

Be sure to drink at least two cups of water within three hours of exercising. Once you start your workout, try to drink about a cup of water every fifteen minutes. Keep on drinking once you're done. Drink another 8 ounces within a half-hour of finishing your workout [2].

Drinking Alcohol? Follow It Up with a Glass of Water

Like coffee and tea, alcohol is dehydrating. Instead of following up a martini with another one, make it a tall glass of water. You're more likely to stay hydrated, you'll save yourself from the extra calories of another drink, and you'll help get rid of toxic by-products from the alcohol [2].

Lost Count? Check Your Urine

If you can't remember how many cups of water you've had today, take a look at the color of your urine. If you're well hydrated, it should be pale yellow, Hawley says. If it's darker, keep drinking [1].

What Counts As Water?

Obviously, plain old water is a perfect way to fill your stomach and give your body the hydration it needs without ingesting a single calorie. But what about the other drinks we like to fill our cups with?

Caffeine from black tea and coffee can dehydrate you, so they're not the best choices for getting to your daily water goal. Juice, sweetened iced tea, and soda are packed with calories. (And diet soda, teas, and juices may make you crave sweets.)

Here are some smart choices.

- Nonfat or low-fat milk
- Fruit juice in moderation
- Vegetable juice
- Teas that contain no or very little caffeine, such as green, chamomile, orange blossom, white, oolong, and many more. (Tip: Brew a cup of hot tea and pour it over ice for a healthy glass of iced tea.)
- Sparkling water, which you can flavor yourself with fruit (such as lemon and lime, and let it sit overnight in the fridge), or buy naturally flavored sparkling waters that contain no sugar sweeteners
- Broth or broth-based soups, such as vegetable soup

A Definite Drink No-No: Super-Sweet Coffee Drinks

There are plenty of people who can't start their day without a cup of coffee, and there's nothing wrong with that [8].

Although coffee can be dehydrating, there's nothing wrong with sipping a cup of joe as long as you follow it up with plenty of water. Although coffee has been considered a bad habit in the past, it has actually been found to have no negative effect on health and may actually be good for you [8].

Researchers from Harvard School of Public Health looked at the coffee drinking habits of 130,000 people who participated in the Nurses' Health Study and the Health Professionals Follow-Up study. Drinking coffee had no effect on mortality rates, including deaths from cancer or cardiovascular disease. Other studies suggest that coffee may offer protection from type 2 diabetes, Parkinson's disease, liver cirrhosis, and liver cancer [8].

But here's a cup of coffee to say no to: the ubiquitous sweetened coffee drinks (hot and cold) that are being sold everywhere from Starbucks to McDonald's. Black coffee has zero calories. Add a splash of nonfat milk and you're up to only about 15 or 20 calories [5]. But order a 24-ounce Frappuccino at Starbucks with whole milk and whipped cream, and you'll down around 500 calories, depending on the flavor [8, 9].

Then, Get Water from Your Food

As you're sipping water from your cup, it's also important to be sure you're getting plenty of water in your food. Water boosts the weight and volume of your food without adding calories, so you can eat more and feel more satisfied for dramatically fewer calories than if you ate more calorie-dense foods.

For example, eat ten luscious grapes, and you'll get only 34 satisfying calories. If you ate the same weight (1.7 ounces) of raisins, on the other hand, you'd get 144 calories [5].

Research has clearly shown that when people sit down to a large portion of food, they're going to eat it. So why not fill your plate with big portions of food that help foster weight loss—vegetables, in particular, which are naturally high in water [11]?

Barbara Rolls, PhD, has conducted several studies that show that eating foods low in energy density is a key factor in feeling satisfied on fewer calories and losing weight [11].

One study found that eating a low-energy-dense (low-calorie) salad before a main course of pasta resulted in eating fewer calories during the meal, especially when the salad was larger. The key was eating the foods that were less energy dense at the start of the meal [11].

In another study, sixty men and women ate lunch at the researchers' laboratory once a week for five weeks and were served soup followed by a meal. Eating soup before the meal significantly lowered the amount of calories they ate for the entire meal, compared to eating no soup [12].

Water-rich and fiber-rich foods are high on the list of low-energy-density foods [12]. You learned in Chapter 12 how to increase fiber in your diet. Here's how to increase water-rich foods.

Make a Habit of Starting with Soup, Salad, or Veggies

Follow the lead of the research studies and start your meal with the healthy, high-volume, low-calorie foods that will give you satisfaction [12].

Supersize the Healthy Way

If you usually have an omelet in the morning, add in vegetables such as spinach, broccoli, or green peppers to get more satisfaction from your morning meal. (You might find you need fewer high-calorie foods, such as cheese in your omelet, when you do.) The same can be done when you're making baked ziti, lasagna, pizza, soups, chili, casseroles, and plenty of other dishes [12].

Have Plenty of High-Water Foods at the Ready

Keep fresh and frozen fruits and vegetables—including salad ingredients and soup that you can stock in the freezer—so you always have satisfying foods that will help you lose weight [12].

When You Want to Splurge, Consider a High-Volume, Lower-Calorie Splurge

Fat-free chocolate pudding has just 100 calories a serving, while an extra large chocolate bar delivers 230 calories, but the pudding weighs more and will feel more satisfying in your stomach [12].

It's a dieter's dream come true. When it comes to the foods above, eat big portions and you'll still lose weight.

What Works for Me

Carol Brannan, therapeutic body worker in Eureka, CA

You could say that I've experienced the full spectrum when it comes to weight and dieting. I started out as a young child being pretty obese. Both of my parents were alcoholics, and I used food for comfort and security. By the time I was around twelve years old I weighed 110 pounds. (As an adult, I'm only four-feet-ten-inches tall, so that was a high weight for my small frame).

I was teased incessantly in school, which I hated. In an effort to lose weight, I went in the complete opposite direction and developed anorexia nervosa. I restricted food so severely that my weight fell to under forty pounds, and I ended up in a coma for a couple of days.

My family was Roman Catholic and my mother went to church every day I was in the hospital to light a candle for me, but the candle wouldn't stay lit. She thought it was a sign that I wasn't going to survive. But miraculously, I did survive. I was very sick for a year and spent two or three years in recovery, but I managed to get to a healthy weight and stay there.

I did it by learning to redirect my energy from being a perfect anorexic to a perfect healthy person. I started thinking of food as fuel and medicine for my body. Eating healthy has been a focus for the majority of my life.

I'm fifty-seven now, and over the years I've tried almost every diet out there. I tried a carb-loading diet in the seventies, a low-glycemic diet, volumetrics (eating high-volume, low-density foods), food combining, gluten-free, the body ecology diet, the blood-type diet, and more.

And for the last thirty years I've been a vegetarian with on and off periods of being a strict vegan. However, today I have started eating animal products again for health reasons.

I think it helped that I had an open mind to all different ways of eating, and when I tried a diet, I picked elements from it that worked for me that I continued even after moving on to another way of eating.

I have learned to eat whole foods instead of processed foods, high-fiber foods, and high-volume foods. I have also learned that drinking plenty of water, especially before meals, really fills me up. Today, I eat 100 percent organic and nothing processed. Very few of my foods come out of a box or a bag. Almost everything I eat I make from scratch, because I think it's the healthiest way to live.

Today I'm a healthy one hundred pounds for my height. In the past, I might have been stricter about the way I ate, but today my eating is a more intuitive and gentle process.

(continued)

(continued)

I consider myself a recovered food addict. I don't think it's something that can be cured, because we can't abstain totally from food. What you can do is to redirect your energy from abusing food to something healthier. I went from food being my ultimate comfort to being my ultimate enemy to now being my friend.

One Caveat to Drinking Lots of Water

As with everything in life, you can get too much of a good thing, even when it comes to drinking water. Do some research on water and you'll read references to water intoxication and warnings not to drink too much because it could lead to death [4].

The good news is that water intoxication is very rare and you need to drink quite a bit of water in just a short period of time to do damage. When researchers examined military cases of water intoxication (including three deaths), they found that they happened when people drank more than five liters (often ten to twenty liters) in a few hours [9].

Too much water leads to a condition called hyponatremia [9]. When there's not enough sodium around the cells, water floods the body's cells for balance, but that makes the cells swell. It's dangerous when that happens to brain cells, which don't have room to expand, and that leads to confusion and hallucinations and can even cause a loss of consciousness, coma, and death [10].

Water intoxication can happen when you're exerting yourself in intense heat and drink much too much water. It's extremely important to stay hydrated in those conditions, but to be safe limit your fluid intake to one to one and a half liters an hour [9].

The Take-Home Message

When you keep your water consumption within the right range, you can see big results on the scale. Hawley works with obese patients who are preparing for gastric bypass surgery by eating a healthy diet, exercising, and focusing on getting plenty of fluids. Just focusing on water before surgery has made a huge difference in some of their lives.

"I know people who lost eighty to one hundred pounds just focusing on drinking plenty of no-calorie water and not confusing thirst with hunger," she says.

It couldn't be simpler: Drink plenty of water—for your health and your waistline.

📖 Dietitian's Diary

Hydration How-Tos

Here are a few things you should know to help you stay healthy and hydrated.

Alcohol and Caffeine

In short, they both dehydrate and, when mixed together, they combine their efforts. Alcohol is usually mixed with another fluid that helps hydrate. But a caffeinated soda and liquor mix is a dehydrating concoction of alcohol and caffeine. This is because alcohol and caffeine are both diuretics, so when we mix them with another liquid, such as ice or soda water, it makes us run to the restroom and dehydrate.

Alcohol also breaks down the glycogen stored by our liver and expels it in our urine. Combine these two effects (with various other metabolic reactions), and you have a hangover. Drinking a glass/bottle of water between each adult libation will help rid your body of the toxic by-products of your imbibing. Drinking water will also help decrease the overall amount of alcohol you drink by

🎗 TIPS

Always hydrate. Keep a water bottle with you. Figure out how much water your bottle holds and divide your fluid needs by the holding volume [13]. Now you know how many times you have to fill your bottle. During a nontraining day, drink at least five 16-ounce water bottles a day (80 ounces total).

Water can get boring. Some calorie-free ways of adding flavor would be adding a slice of lemon, lime, or cucumber to your water, or try some fresh herbs, such as mint or basil. I take a few mint leaves, tear them in quarters to release all the essential oils, and put them into a tea infuser. I put the leaves into a tea ball so I don't have to fish the leaves out later or get them stuck in my teeth. Let the leaves sit in the cold water a few minutes and remove.

There are always caffeine-free teas if the water tricks don't quite do it for you. Making your own iced tea lets you control the amount of sugar, if any, in your beverage. Get fruit-flavored bags of tea, such as peach or apple. Take about four bags of tea to a pitcher of super hot water (just before boiling is best). Let the bags steep for about five minutes, depending on how strong you like your tea, and then discard the bags. Chill tea in the fridge and sip over ice. Hydrating and tasty.

putting a cold nonalcoholic drink in your hand for awhile. Pellegrino is just as cool and refreshing as a vodka and soda.

Exercise

It's especially important to consume enough fluid when you're exercising. Dehydration can cause poor performance and lead to fatigue, cardiovascular stress, and increased risk of heat illness [14].

You need to consume additional fluid throughout the day when exercising. In the three hours prior to your workout or event, drink two cups of water. During your event, drink about a cup of water every fifteen minutes. This will be a 16-ounce bottle of water for every thirty minutes on the treadmill. Postevent, drink to replenish any weight lost during exercise. Forgot to weigh yourself before your workout? Just keep drinking! Drink 8 ounces within thirty minutes after exercise and 16 ounces for every pound of weight lost during exercise [15].

Where do all the sports drinks come in? For exercise that is less than sixty minutes of moderate intensity, water is a good choice. It is when we have long (more than sixty minutes) and/or intense (for any duration) activity that sports drinks are helpful for replenishing our bodies with electrolytes, fluids, and carbohydrates. If your exercise is not long or intense, try to avoid the extra calories. Besides sports drinks, watery foods such as fruits and vegetables also help replace potassium lost in exercise. Sodium losses can be replaced with vegetable juice or broth-based soups. I eat a piece of fruit on my way out of the gym.

Recipes

KICK UP YOUR GLASS OF WATER

Most of the day you should be sipping water to get enough fluids, but that doesn't mean what's in your cup has to bore you to death. Try dropping one or more of these flavor boosters into your glass or a pitcher of water to get more satisfaction from your drink.

- Lemon slices
- Lime rounds
- Orange wedges
- Strawberry halves
- Blackberries, slightly crushed
- Melon or cantaloupe chunks
- Watermelon squares
- Mango chunks
- Peach slices

- Cucumber rounds
- Celery sticks
- Fresh mint leaves
- Fresh basil leaves
- Fresh, peeled ginger slivers

TRY THESE GREAT COMBOS:

- Cantaloupe and cucumber
- Lemon and cucumber
- Lemon and lime
- Mint and lime
- Basil and strawberries

Satisfaction Solution: De-Stress

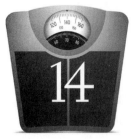

See How De-Stressing Helps You Achieve Your Weight-Loss Goals

Remember the classic 1980 Calgon commercial for bubble bath? A picture of bumper-to-bumper traffic, an angry boss, a crying child, and a dirty dog swirl around a woman until she cries, "Calgon, take me away!" [1].

Today, you could add a beeping cell phone, an overstuffed e-mail inbox, a computer that's on the fritz (because, at five years old, it's *ancient*), extreme work demands, high unemployment rates, and an economy that doesn't look like it's getting better any time soon.

What does all of that have to do with the size of your waistband? A whole lot.

Stress plays a huge role in weight gain and the inability to lose weight, says Amy Wood, PsyD.

"When life gets stressful, it's hard to make good decisions and use self-discipline, and often the first thing that goes is healthful eating," she says. "You reach for food as a quick-fix stress reducer, and usually the foods that provide that quick fix aren't healthful."

There are also complex processes going on to increase your hunger and cause you to gain weight. In a recent animal study, researchers put rats under social stress by putting them in colonies where one dominant male became the leader. The subordinate rats under ate while in the colonies, but when they were moved to live individually and were able to eat freely, they overate compared to a group of rats that hadn't been exposed to social stress. They ate fewer times a day, but when they did eat, they ate big meals [2].

As a result, the rats that had been exposed to stress gained weight, particularly belly fat [2]. Experts say stress also has that effect on people, causing them to overeat and put on weight around their middle [3].

215

On top of weight gain, stress may also increase risk for depression, heart disease, digestive trouble, sleep issues, and memory problems and can exacerbate skin conditions like eczema [4].

It's no surprise that stress is bad for you. It sure feels bad when you're right in the middle of it. And it might feel like trying to deal with stress is a losing battle. But the truth is you have more control over your body's reaction to life's roller coaster than you might think.

Why Stress Sends the Scale Skyrocketing

Some people lose weight when they're under stress, while others gain. If you tend to see the scale rise when you're under stress, here are a couple of reasons why.

Emotional Eating

When you feel intense, uncomfortable emotions, such as frustration, anger, fear, confusion, or impatience, it's much harder to stay on track toward healthful, disciplined living, Dr. Wood says. Stress can cause so much emotional distress that you reach for a quick fix, which may be a big bowl of macaroni and cheese or a cigarette or a beer [5]. (If you need a refresher on emotional eating, go back to Chapter 2.)

Depression may also be a factor. People who are obese often deal with depression as well, especially women. One study found that women who were obese had a 37 percent greater chance of suffering from major depression. It's like a never-ending cycle: You feel bad about your body and/or your health, and that leads to overeating, which leads to a bump on the scale, and that can lead to more depression, and the cycle starts all over again [6].

Also, binge eating can be a symptom of depression. Research has found that 51 percent of binge eaters had suffered from major depression. And if you're a woman who was a binge eater and then was teased about the way you looked, you have a strong chance of not being satisfied with your body and developing depression [6].

Stress Hormones

We're hard wired with a life saving "fight or flight" response to danger. When faced with a threat—ages ago, that meant coming across a wild animal, like a bear—our bodies release the stress hormones adrenaline and cortisol.

Adrenaline gets your heart racing, pushes your blood pressure up, and gives you energy to fight or flee. Cortisol causes your blood sugar to surge, helps your brain use the blood sugar, and gets your body ready to repair from injuries. It also changes your immune responses and inhibits digestion, your reproductive system, and growth—all while working with parts of your brain that influence your mood, feelings of fear, and your motivation. When danger is gone, your body goes back to a normal state [4].

That works really well if you're in a dire situation and you're fighting or running for your life. The problem is that today we experience emotional stress that causes the same reactions in the body several times a day. And when we're talking about work stress or traffic jams or having a to-do list that feels like it could reach the moon, we don't have the option of fighting or fleeing—we have to stick it out [7].

What does that have to do with your weight? Research has found that circulating cortisol levels trigger an increase in belly fat, which is the type of fat that puts you at greater risk for diabetes and heart disease. A Yale study of fifty-nine women found that those who had more belly fat (even if they were normal weight) were more vulnerable to stress and cortisol compared to women who had smaller waists [8, 3].

What to Do in the Moment

We may never have to run for our lives from a wild animal (if we're lucky), but we're certainly not lacking in stress today. A 2010 survey by the American Psychological Association found that most Americans feel pretty darned stressed. The majority surveyed rated their stress as being moderate to high. Two-fifths of those surveyed said they overeat or choose unhealthy foods when they're under stress [9].

When you're feeling stressed—because you just received some unsettling news or you have too much to do and too little time, or you're listening to talk radio again and you're getting fired up—try one or more of these strategies for immediate calm.

- Take some deep breaths and slow down your breathing (try the Dirga breaths described in Chapter 15) [10].
- Count to ten [10].
- Head outside and get some sunshine. One study suggests that people who work outside in the wintertime in Denmark have fewer mood problems than people who don't work outside [11].
- Go for a walk, work in the garden, play basketball, wash your car, practice your kickboxing moves, or get your body moving in any way you choose [12].

- Do a little tai chi, which has been called "meditation in motion." The gentle exercise and stretching force you to slow down and feel more calm [13].

- Take a few minutes to meditate, in which you focus on breathing and let go of each thought that pops into your head.

- Listen to calming music. It's proven to relieve stress [14].

- Strike a few relaxing yoga poses (such as the ones described in Chapter 15). One study found that women who regularly do hatha yoga recover from stress more quickly than women who are new to yoga [15].

- Visualize something that's calming to you, including the smells, sights, noises, sounds, and feel of the place, whether it's at the ocean or deep in the woods [16].

- Watch a funny video online (keep those bookmarked for when you need them) or thumb through a book of jokes to let yourself laugh.

Long-Term Stress-Busting Strategies

The rest of the time, there's still plenty you can do to overcome stress, and it's worth the effort. Experts say you can't be successful at weight loss if you're bogged down with negative emotions or stress [6]. Take the time now to put a lid on stress so you can reach your goals.

Recognize Your Stress Signs

You may have a hard time concentrating when you're stressed, whereas someone else might get headaches. If you can recognize your body's reaction to stress at the first signs, you can do something about it before you find yourself devouring an entire pizza [17].

Keep Your Meals Balanced

You might be craving a big bowl of pasta when you're under stress, but eating carbs can actually increase the amount of cortisol in your system. Researchers fed ten men shakes around lunchtime for four days and measured their cortisol levels before eating and for three hours after eating. When the men were given a shake that contained fat or protein, concentrations of cortisol dropped significantly, the study said. But when the men were given shakes that contained carbohydrates, their cortisol levels were higher [18]. This is another reason to be sure you're getting enough protein.

Sweat a Little—On a Regular Basis

Exercise is a well-known stress buster. It releases endorphins and neurotransmitters in your brain that make you feel good, lower the number of immune system chemicals that can contribute to depression, and literally warm your body temperature, which is calming [9].

At the same time, it's the perfect way to clear your mind and think about something besides what's bothering you. And when you're done with your workout, you'll probably feel more self-confident and better about yourself [12].

Recruit Others

Rather than relying on your own willpower to pass up your kids' Pop-Tarts, make your kitchen a junk-food-free zone and explain to your family why it's important to you. Your family's health will benefit, and you'll feel less stress when foods you tend to overeat are out of the house [6].

And while you're at it, garner support from outside of your family by asking friends to join you in trying to lose weight and exercise. Maybe this is a good time to check out an Overeaters Anonymous meeting or another support group that you find through your local hospital or school [6].

Designate Time for Decompressing

Even if it's just ten minutes, take time to do something that makes you feel calm every day. Meditate, do some deep breathing, take a walk, slip into a bubble bath, listen to music, or do something else you enjoy that helps relax you [19].

Unplug

You can't help being plugged in while you're at work, but when you don't have to be, turn off your cell phone and give your computer a rest. Don't let work stress seep into your time at home or on vacation [20].

By All Means, Say No

You'll feel less stress and be able to set yourself up for weight loss when you take charge of your life, Dr. Wood says. We're pulled in a hundred different directions, with responsibilities and requests for our time, but it's important to set limits.

Bring into your life only what feels right, she says. You'll feel more balanced and healthy and be able to ultimately achieve a weight that feels good [5].

Shed Some Positive Light on the Situation

Buried in a mountain of work at your job? Rather than thinking, "I can't do this," tell yourself that you're going to do your best. Negative thoughts add to your stress, but replacing them with positive views can help keep stress under control [10]. If you have a difficult time with this, you might turn to *The Power of Positive Thinking*, by Norman Vincent Peale.

What Works for Me

Tracy Jones, national account manager at Sysco in West Jordan, UT

A few years ago, I was caught up in a vicious cycle of losing and then gaining weight. I'm an avid cyclist, and I would train with my dad for century rides, which are one hundred miles long. But once the rides were over and winter came, I would be less active and gain weight.

Then I had a two-year span where I was down on myself and didn't want to try anything to lose weight. But in January 2010, with the nudging of a friend, I got back into the swing of things. I started doing *20 Second Fitness* exercises, which involved doing twenty seconds of high-intensity exercises (such as fast jumping jacks or high knees) followed by ten seconds of rest. I started doing the exercises for just four minutes and built up to doing them for twelve. Because they were so short, it was easy to do them six days a week.

I was feeling better about myself, and my body was shrinking because my clothes were looser. But after two months of doing the workouts (without changing my diet much), the scale didn't move. I was frustrated, but I kept on doing it every day, having faith that sooner or later the pieces would fit into place. I even brought the DVDs with me on business trips.

Finally, after about two and a half months, my weight started dropping, and it kept going until I had lost more than eighty pounds around month nine.

I also started paying attention to my portions and worked on eating healthier. I like to splurge on chocolate, but instead of buying a big bag of M&Ms, I'd buy a small, fun-size bag.

Diet had some impact on my weight, but I'd say it was really the exercise that did it for me. I know that if I don't move I'm going to gain weight, and it was exercise that got me over a plateau around month six. When the scale wouldn't move anymore, someone told me I had to start working harder, so I did. I kept doing the exercises, and I started really pushing myself.

I enjoy exercise even more now that I'm eighty pounds lighter, and I'm able to do things I never did before. Since losing weight, I've done five century rides, two triathlons, and mud runs, which are races with obstacles.

Whenever I need motivation, I look at my old pictures and the clothes I used to wear, and I know I don't ever want to be there again. That keeps me lacing up my sneakers and heading out the door for a good workout.

Make Sleep a Priority

When you're sleep deprived, your cortisol levels spike, and other hormones that regulate your appetite—leptin and ghrelin—will make you hungry. Aim to get enough sleep so that you can wake up easily and you're not overtired during the day, which is typically seven to nine hours a night for most people [21]. (For much more about sleep, go to Chapter 15.)

When You Have a Bad Day, Let It Go

There's no point in letting a bad day of making poor health choices turn into a bad week. Wake up the next morning to a new day and vow to make it a good day [6].

Don't Give Up

Stress isn't something to tackle just today, this week, or this month. Developing healthy habits to manage stress can help you for years to come and help you keep your weight in check [5].

"To achieve and sustain a healthy weight, you have to lead a balanced life comprised of sufficient sleep, nourishing and satisfying food, enjoyable downtime, positive social support, etc.—all on a regular, ongoing basis," Dr. Wood says [5].

Sometimes Stress-Relief Requires a Self-Inventory

Lowering your stress level might be a bigger project than taking a bubble bath and spending time with friends. Sometimes it means taking the plunge and making life changes [5].

"The Number One way to reduce stress is to take a step back from your life and ask if it's truly the life you want to live," Dr. Wood says. "In this fast-paced world, it's hard to take time out and ask important questions, like, am I really happy with my job, partner, self, or where I live?" [5]

Dr. Wood has seen people who are exasperated that they can't lose weight. But she soon realizes that they've put too much emphasis on losing weight and have neglected the important areas of their lives that need to be in place before they can start losing weight [5].

"I advise these clients to put weight loss on the back burner for awhile and tend to improving other areas of life, such as de-cluttering their house, looking for a new job, improving their relationships, finding healthy ways to increase self-esteem, ending unhealthy situations, becoming more assertive, getting to bed earlier, getting out of debt, and so on," she says [5].

When you start nurturing these areas of your life that need attending to, you'll feel less stress and have more energy to tackle weight loss [5].

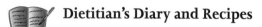 Dietitian's Diary and Recipes

New Comfort Foods

When we are stressed, the first type of food we typically turn to is our mainstay: comfort foods. This is usually because it tastes good and reminds us of a simpler and relaxing time in our lives. My comfort foods often remind me of times where I have triumphed. Scones and vanilla lattes are not only tasty but remind me of my perseverance in finishing college. Chicken fried steak and gravy reminds me of my travels in the South during military training.

Comfort foods are about comfort, not counting calories. But there's no reason comfort foods have to be unhealthy. By this point in the book, you have learned how to successfully decrease the unhealthy fats and unneeded calories from everyday recipes and food choices. Whatever makes your comfort foods your own, make them part of your healthy eating plan in one of two ways: use that meal as your every-once-in-awhile meal and eat smaller portions, or make the recipe healthier.

Here are some of the most popular comfort foods and how to make them a little healthier:

Macaroni and Cheese

- Decrease the amount of cheese used to melt
- Use a low-fat milk cheese
- Try some vegan cheese
- Add vegetables, such as spinach or peas to the recipe
- Use whole-wheat pasta
- For boxed mac 'n' cheese, make the low-fat recipe listed on the box (less butter and nonfat milk)

Chicken Pot Pie

- Add extra vegetables
- Decrease the amount of fat used in the cream sauce by using fat-free milk or soy milk

Chili Mac

- Use whole-wheat pasta
- Add vegetables or more tomatoes
- Decrease amount of fat by using less meat or vegetarian meat substitutes such as Boca Ground Crumbles or Quorn Grounds

Meatloaf and Meatballs

- Add finely diced vegetables
- Substitute some meat with cooked lentils, TVP, or bulgur wheat

Chicken Fried Steak and Gravy

- Use nonfat milk or soy milk to make gravy
- Use less gravy of original recipe with the Fork Method (don't pour gravy over steak)
- Bake the steak instead of deep frying it
- Use a high-fiber side dish, such as wild rice, to help with your Satisfaction Solution

Homemade Cream Soups

- Replace or use less heavy cream and replace needed amount of fluid with fat-free milk or soy milk
- If your recipes include vegetables, then add more

French Fries

- Cut your own potatoes and cook in the oven
- Season with Mrs. Dash Garlic and Herb
- When potatoes are cooked, place under broiler for a couple minutes to crisp up!

Pudding

- Make pudding with nonfat milk or soy milk
- Find a tofu mousse or pudding recipe for a rich snack

Sweet Potato Casserole

- Decrease the amount of butter and sugar in your recipe
- Replace most or all of butter with canola oil
- Don't skimp too much on the marshmallows; ten mini-marshmallows have only 22 calories

Satisfaction Solution: Sleep

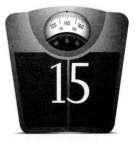

Discover Why Getting Your Zzz's Must Be Part of Your Weight-Loss Plan

What happens when you're doing everything right—you're planning healthy meals, you're cooking and eating the right foods, you're eating at regular intervals throughout the day, you're exercising regularly, you're working on emotional eating—but you still feel the urge to empty a bag of cookies into your mouth?

It might not have to do with what you're putting on your plate. Believe it or not, it might have to do with how much time you're spending putting your head on a pillow [1, 2].

Sleep is as important to your body as breathing, and when you don't get enough it can have far-reaching psychological and physical effects, including weight gain [2].

And yet a shocking number of people don't get enough. When Robert Oexman, DC, director of the Sleep to Live Institute in Joplin, Missouri, gives seminars he asks the people in the room how many get just six hours of sleep a night. "A third of people in the room raise their hands," he says [1].

But that might be part of the reason Americans tend to pack on the pounds. In a six-year study of 276 adults, researchers found that sleeping only five to six hours a night made people 35 percent more likely to gain up to eleven pounds over six years, compared with people who slept seven to eight hours a night [2, 3].

People who slept longer than average—nine to ten hours a night—also gained an average of 3.5 pounds, but a later analysis of sleep studies didn't confirm that sleeping longer affected risk for obesity [2, 3].

In addition to obesity, not getting enough sleep is also associated with other health problems, including diabetes and heart disease [2].

If you're serious about losing weight, you'll make it a point to turn in at a decent hour every night [1]. Consider why sleep is so essential to your weight-loss plan and how to pull off getting more of it every night.

How Sleep Affects Appetite: It's About Hormones

First of all, it's hard to stay motivated to eat healthy and exercise when you're dragging yourself through the day from lack of sleep. But there's more to the story than that. Lack of sleep affects those hormones we talked about in Chapter 1 that affect how hungry you feel. The result: a constant craving for food when you're sleep-deprived, Oexman says [1].

One researcher, Eve Van Cauter, PhD, has found that just six days of sleeping just four hours a night leads to changes in the body that bring on a prediabetic state. She has also found that people who go on just four hours of sleep a night for six days want to eat more and more even after they should already be full [2].

Hormones that regulate appetite are at play. Leptin levels, which let you know when you're full, go down when your sleep is restricted. Ghrelin, the hormone that stimulates your appetite, increases when you don't get enough sleep [2].

Meanwhile, the stress hormone cortisol skyrockets when you're sleep deprived, and higher cortisol levels can lead to insulin resistance, which raises the risk of obesity and diabetes [2].

When researchers restrict people's sleep, they end up with a pretty insatiable appetite. Researchers took in eleven people for two 14-day stays in a sleep lab. They were allowed either 8.5 or only 5.5 hours of sleep a night and could eat as much food as they wanted during the day. When their sleep was restricted, they ate 221 to 283 more calories a day in snacks than when they got more sleep [4].

How Much Do You Need?

When you skimp on sleep, the odds of being able to lose weight and maintain a healthy weight are stacked against you. For your health and your weight, get enough sleep.

So, how much is enough? Sleep experts say the average adult needs seven to nine hours of sleep a night (adolescents and children need more.) [2].

But remember, seven to nine is an average. Some people may need a little bit more, Oexman says. When you wake up easily in the morning and you're alert throughout the day (without using caffeine to stay awake), you're getting enough sleep, he says [1].

How to Sneak in Some Extra Sleep

A 2011 National Sleep Foundation poll found that most Americans get a little under seven hours of sleep on weeknights, on average, and that two-thirds of people say they're not getting enough during the week [5].

Sleep is not beyond your reach. Take these steps and you'll be waking up feeling refreshed—and maybe even a little lighter.

Stick with Your Daily Exercise Routine

As long as you're not exercising in the few hours before going to sleep, the activity should help you sleep better [2].

Watch Your Caffeine and Alcohol Intake

Drinking caffeine can affect your sleep for up to twelve hours, so try to limit your coffee, tea, and sodas to earlier in the day.

And while alcohol may make you drowsy and fall asleep, your sleep will be disrupted as your body metabolizes the drinks [2].

Finish Dinner Two to Three Hours Before Bed

Your body's core temperature falls when it's time to go to sleep, but food digestion causes your core temperature to go up. That means it's hard to fall asleep if you've eaten too close to bedtime [2].

Stay on a Regular Sleep Schedule

Try to go to bed and wake up at the same time every day, including on weekends. When your schedule changes it can disrupt your circadian rhythm, which influences sleeping and waking [2].

Start a Healthy Pre-Bedtime Ritual

People tend to spend the hour before going to bed watching television or on the computer. But one of your body's cues for falling asleep is a decrease in the amount of light, Oexman says. You can prime your body for sleep by lowering the lights, turning off the television and computer, and spending thirty to sixty minutes before bed in a dim environment as you prepare for bed, he says [1].

Sleep rituals can help wind you down for a restful night, too. Take a warm bath, read a book, or listen to soft music as you get ready for bed [6]. What not to do: get yourself fired up by watching the news, reading about politics, or watching an action-packed movie [2].

Put Away Distractions

We simply have too many distractions today that keep us up later than we should be. You're already turning off the television and computer in the hours before bed. It's also time to turn off your cell phone, put the Kindle away, and resist playing one more game of Angry Birds on your iTouch device [1].

And don't even keep a television, computer, or cell phone in your bedroom. Your bedroom should be a calming environment that fosters restful sleep [1].

Turn Down the Thermostat

Your body is programmed to go to sleep when it's chilly and wake up when it's warm, so setting your room temperature to between sixty-eight and seventy degrees at night will keep you at a comfortable sleeping temperature under the covers [2].

Climb into Bed in Darkness

Even small amounts of light can decrease your melatonin level, a hormone that regulates your sleep. Turn off the light in your room, use room-darkening shades if it's still light at bedtime, and even turn your alarm clock away from you or put a towel over it if it lights up, Oexman says [1].

Avoid Naps

Napping during the day can lead to having trouble sleeping at night. If you really need a nap, don't sleep more than forty-five minutes [2].

Get Help for Sleep Disorders

If you think you have a sleep disorder, such as insomnia or sleep apnea, go to a sleep lab to get evaluated and treated if needed [2]. Getting better sleep can help you feel so good that you're more motivated to lose weight. And when you lose just 10 percent of your weight, problems like sleep apnea become less severe and you sleep better [7].

Turn Off the Chatter and Go to Sleep

Even when your external environment is primed for sleep and you've gotten yourself into bed early enough, a racing mind can get in the way of rest.

"Very often, at the end of the day you're going over what happened during that day," says Sheila Abrahams, a yoga instructor in Hernando, Florida, and adjunct professor of nutrition at College of Central Florida [8].

That chattering mind keeps you from falling asleep, Abrahams says. But there are ways to put an end to ruminating thoughts that are keeping you awake and let go of stress and tension your body is holding on to. Yoga, meditation, guided relaxation, acupuncture, and biofeedback all await to help you get a good night's rest and get your body burning fat.

As we mentioned, if you're having chronic sleep problems, see a physician first to rule out serious diseases such as sleep apnea. Once you've ruled out serious problems, turning to these strategies can do wonders for your nights [8].

Yoga

If you've been to a few yoga classes at the gym, you're familiar with yoga poses. However, postures are just one branch of yoga, Abrahams says. There are actually eight branches of classical yoga, including postures, breath control, and meditations [8].

All three parts of yoga—the breathing, the postures, and meditation—can help you get a better night's sleep because yoga invokes a relaxation response, Abrahams says. It's the opposite of the body's fight-or-flight response to stress, and that helps you withdraw from the sensory overload that may be keeping you awake [8]. Here's what to do:

Relaxing Dirga Pranayama, or Three-Part Breathing

1. Lie on the floor, flat on your back.
2. Inhale deeply through your nose.
3. Fill your belly with breath, expanding it like a balloon.
4. Exhale by expelling the air from your belly, through your nose.
5. Repeat two to three times.
6. On your next exhale, fill your belly first, then draw in a little more air and let it expand into the rib cage.
7. Exhale air first from your rib cage, then the belly.
8. Repeat for two or three breaths

9. On the next inhale, fill your belly, then your rib cage, then your upper chest.

10. On your exhale, let the air go from your upper chest, then your rib cage, then your belly.

11. Repeat for two or three breaths.

And if you're still not relaxed ...

Try Alternate-Nostril Breathing

Yoga embraces yin and yang, so alternating between breathing out of each nostril can have a wonderfully calming effect because it balances the mind, Abrahams says [8].

Do this as you sit upright in your bed at night before going to sleep:

- Start with a Dirga breath by inhaling and exhaling.

- On the next inhale, close off your right nostril with your thumb and inhale through your left nostril.

- Take your thumb away and exhale through your right nostril while closing off the left nostril with your ring finger.

- Remove your ring finger and exhale through your left nostril while closing off your right nostril with your thumb again.

- Repeat for one to ten minutes [8].

Get into a Relaxing Pose

You don't want to choose just any yoga pose to help you go to sleep, because some are invigorating, whereas others relax you. Abrahams recommends these relaxing and restorative poses for better sleep. You don't need a yoga mat; a carpeted floor will work just fine [8].

Focus on breathing while you do each of these poses, and hold each for thirty seconds to a minute. If you feel any type of pain, get out of the pose immediately [8].

- **Balasana (child's pose):** On the floor, kneel in a position with your forehead on the floor, your behind resting on your heels, and your arms either stretched out in front of you or at your sides [8].

- **Downward-facing dog:** Get on your hands and knees, with your knees below your hips and your hands in front of your shoulders. Inhale, and as you exhale straighten your legs and press your hips up so that you form the shape of a triangle with the floor. Press your heels down as you do it, but it's not necessary for them to reach the floor (Note: if you have severe high blood pressure or you're pregnant, inverted poses like this one aren't recommended.) [8].

- If you have carpal tunnel syndrome and you can't put pressure on your hands, try the **dolphin pose**, Abrahams says. Rather than keeping your palms flat on the floor, hold them in fists, or go on your forearms and get the same benefit. [8]

- **Savasana (corpse pose):** In bed, lie on your back with your heels together and your toes out with your arms at your sides. Keep still and practice your Dirga breaths until you fall asleep [8].

Meditation

There are different types of meditation within yoga, but Abrahams recommends going with the simplest form, which invokes the relaxation response [8].

Sit on the floor in a lotus pose, with your legs folded or in a chair with your feet on the ground. Close your eyes and practice Dirga breaths, concentrating on your breath, while you say a mantra, such as "I'm breathing in, I'm breathing out" or "ohm." When thoughts float into your head, let them go without ruminating on them [8].

Guided Relaxation

Another way to go out like a light is to use guided relaxation as you lie in your bed. Lie on your back, and tense each muscle in your body and then relax it before moving on to another muscle. Start with your toes, Abrahams says. Lift your toes slightly and then release them. Then move to your feet, followed by your calves, etc. If you prefer, you can buy guided relaxation CDs or download them from the Internet to listen to while you relax [8].

Acupuncture

Acupuncture has been used for thousands of years in China, and it may be worth a try for insomnia. When you receive acupuncture, a practitioner inserts very thin needles into your skin at certain areas of your body to balance the flow of energy. Some Western practitioners believe the needles stimulate your muscles and nerves to increase blood flow [9].

Evidence that acupuncture can help with insomnia and other sleep problems is mixed, but there are some small studies that suggest it can improve sleep, and it's still an area that researchers are actively pursuing [10, 11].

In one study of people with sleep apnea who weren't able to tolerate the typical treatment for the disease, acupuncture helped foster sleep. When a group of forty patients were either treated with acupuncture or were given sham acupuncture, those who received the legitimate therapy woke up fewer times during the night [12].

What Works for Me

Hoang Uyen X. Nguyen, a coordinator in television advertising traffic, based in Egan, MN

For me, being successful at losing weight is about finding a good reason to do it. It started when my sister got engaged and asked me to be a bridesmaid in her wedding. It was the perfect opportunity to drop some pounds, so she and I started working out together.

We did the Beachbody exercise videos by Tony Horton together, and we logged our progress. Each week we measured our upper arms, busts, waists, hips, and thighs and put them on index cards. That allowed us to track our progress from week to week. Watching those numbers shrink was motivating, and it was great to have a partner along the way.

I also started cutting down the portions of food I had been eating. Instead of digging into a huge bowl of rice, I'd eat a smaller one. Rather than eating two eggs, I'd have one. When I had a sandwich, hamburger, or wrap, I would eat half at my meal and save the other half for later. At restaurants I chose the healthy suggestions listed on the menu and almost always took part of my meal home to have the next day.

On top of that, I tried to be as active as possible. I chose parking spots that were farther away, and I took walks whenever I could. I also love to dance, and I take every opportunity I can to move. I dance around my house, and I go out dancing at nightclubs.

By the time my sister's wedding came, I had lost around fifteen pounds.

I went through the whole process again when my sorority sister got married and asked me to be a bridesmaid. By then I had already been down the road of losing weight, so I just kept the momentum going.

It really helped to have a goal: looking good in those bridesmaid dresses. But now it's about being healthy. Although I think it's good to be happy at whatever weight you are, I feel healthier and better when my weight is down.

Biofeedback

If your insomnia is a result of anxiety and muscle tension, biofeedback may help. An independent panel put together by the National Institutes of Health found that biofeedback can help with sleep problems and treating chronic pain [13].

During treatment, a practitioner will put electrodes on your body that are attached to a machine that measures your stress levels. As you get feedback about your heart rate, blood pressure, and muscle tension, you learn how to have control over your body's reaction to stress. When you're able to recognize tension in your body and work to alleviate it, you'll be able to relax and go to sleep more easily [14].

Sleep is so important to your health and your weight—not to mention your sanity—that it's just not worth it to skip out on it. Before you decide to stay up late watching reruns of Seinfeld, think about the impact it may have on your weight-loss goals [1].

In today's world of constant distraction, that means it's going to take some commitment on your part, Oexman says. Make sleep a priority in your life, and you may just find that the other things you're working toward—wearing an old pair of jeans from your thinner days, finishing a half marathon, fitting in an airplane seat with room to spare—will fall into place [1].

Dietitian's Diary

Sweet Dreams

For most of us, life experiences have shown us that caffeine and alcohol can lead to sleeplessness. But what foods have an opposite effect on our bodies? Most people equate sleepiness with the following items; tryptophan, warm milk, melatonin, and chamomile tea. Let's review these items and their effect on our sleep.

Tryptophan is an amino acid (a building block of protein) that encourages the production of serotonin in the brain. Serotonin is a neurotransmitter that calms us and helps regulate sleep. When we think of our Thanksgiving Day turkey, we think of the tryptophan from the turkey putting us into bloated sleepiness. Surprisingly enough, it is not all Mr. Gobble's fault. Turkey has both tryptophan and tyrosine (an amino acid that helps wake up the brain). If you ate only turkey, the two amino acids would essentially cancel out each other's effect on your brain. It is actually the carbohydrate-rich parts of the meal (those pesky mashed potatoes, yams, stuffing, and cranberries) that stimulate the release of insulin in your body, which clears the bloodstream of the tyrosine. This allows the tryptophan direct access to your brain, triggering serotonin synthesis. This is why, if you eat a meal chock-full of carbohydrates, rather than a balanced meal, you'll feel lethargic [15].

When you were growing up, did your mom ever give you a glass of **warm milk** to help you sleep? There is a reason it works, besides reminding us of the comforts of home. Milk contains both tryptophan and calcium. Calcium and tryptophan work together to create melatonin [15]. Melatonin helps regulate our body's internal clock and plays a part in our sleep patterns [16]. As a little side note, it has not been proven that warm milk creates this effect any more than cold milk.

This brings us to the **melatonin supplement pills**. The National Sleep Foundation claims that there is little to no benefit of taking melatonin pills to improve sleep [17]. Melatonin pills may, however, help you recover from jet lag over several time zones and some insomnia [16]. The University of Maryland Medical Center states that, for insomnia, you should work with your doctor to find a safe and effective dose of melatonin. In general, "1 to 3 mg one hour before bedtime is usually effective, although doses as low as 0.1 to 0.3 mg may improve sleep for some people" [16]. You and your doctor will know you have the right dose when you have restful sleep and little to no daytime fatigue due to lack of sleep. For jet lag, the university states that "0.5 to 5 mg of melatonin one hour prior to bedtime at final destination has been used in several studies. Another approach that has been used is 1 to 5 mg one hour before bedtime for two days prior to departure and for two to three days upon arrival at final destination." Remember to think ahead when it comes to taking melatonin pills for jet lag. You don't want to rent a great convertible and drive it in a fog.

A nice hot cup of **chamomile tea** before bed can be a potent sleep aid. In fact, research indicates that it can be just as effective as the prescription drug benzodiazepine as a sleep aid (when tested on rats) [18]. The Food and Drug Administration considers chamomile to be safe, so enjoy your tea while you wind down from your day.

Recipes

After you've had a good night's sleep, greet the day with these great breakfast recipes:

BREAKFAST FRITTATA   Serves: 5

2 tablespoons olive oil, extra virgin
1 cup red onion, chopped
1 tablespoon garlic, minced
1 red bell pepper
¾ cup celery stalk, chopped
1 fifteen-ounce can cannellini beans, drained and rinsed
4 egg whites
4 eggs
4 tablespoons sesame seeds
Black pepper, fresh ground, to taste

Directions:

1. Whisk together egg white, whole eggs, and pepper. Set aside.

2. Heat oil in a pan of medium depth that is oven safe.

3. Sauté onion, garlic, red pepper, and celery until softened.

4. Turn temperature down to low to medium heat.

5. Stir in beans to combine.

6. Slowly add egg mixture to pan and stir.

7. Do not touch egg mixture. Cook on low to medium heat until the sides of the frittata can easily pull away from the side.

8. Top with sesame seeds.

9. Put under broiler (in oven) until seeds are lightly toasted and the frittata is a light golden brown on top.

Per serving: 253 calories, 13.5 g fat, 17.7 g carbohydrate, 1.1 g fiber, 15.2 g protein.

HONEY PECAN OATMEAL   Serves: 2

1 cup oatmeal, old fashioned
2 oz. pecan halves
2 tablespoons honey

Directions:

1. Cook oats according to package using water as the liquid.

2. Stir in nuts and honey.

3. Serve warm.

Per serving: 426 calories, 21.7 g fat, 49 g carbohydrate, 2.6 g fiber, 8.7 g protein.

PUMPKIN PANCAKES   Serves: 6 pancakes

Dry ingredients:
1 cup buckwheat pancake mix
¼ cup brown sugar
1½ teaspoons baking powder
¼ teaspoon salt
½ teaspoon cinnamon
¼ teaspoon nutmeg

Wet ingredients:
1 teaspoon ginger root, grated
2 medium egg whites
¾ cup soy or nonfat milk
1 cup pumpkin puree
1 teaspoon almond extract

Directions:

1. Combine all dry ingredients in a large bowl.
2. In another bowl, combine wet ingredients.
3. Slowly stir wet ingredients into dry ingredients.
4. Cook in a nonstick pan on low to medium heat on each side for about 2 minutes.

TIP

These pancakes are much denser than you may be used to, so make sure you cook low and slow in order to avoiding burning the pancakes.

Going the Long Haul

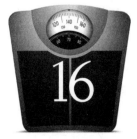

Find Out Why You're Now Ready to Change Your Life

Are you still hungry?

Our guess is that by now you're hungrier for life than you are for food. You're hungry to start living in control.

Hunger isn't something you have to be afraid of anymore. Hunger is a sign that your body is healthy. Hunger means your body is doing what it should, says Keri Gans, RD, author of *The Small-Change Diet* and a nutritionist in private practice in New York City [1].

"We're supposed to be hungry," she says, because it's a sign that it's time to nourish our bodies. When we use hunger signals, along with signals of satiety, as our guide, we're on the right track for weight loss [1].

We're not supposed to be famished. When you're famished, you can't think rationally about what you should eat [1].

And we're not supposed to be overstuffed. Some people think they need more food to hold them over because they're afraid of getting hungry later, but that only undermines your goals [1].

If you have a plan for eating; and you've stocked your fridge with nutritious, satisfying foods; and you know what you'll do when you're eating outside of the house, hunger doesn't have to be in control.

When that happens, it will be easier to stick with healthy eating for life.

It's also important to remember that a healthy life is one of balance. Choose healthy foods the majority of the time, but know that you don't have to be 100 percent perfect, Gans says [1].

When you allow yourself the foods you enjoy, you're less likely to overeat. Gans goes to dinner every Saturday night and doesn't hesitate to indulge in a piece of chocolate cake that she shares with her husband. "I can have four or five bites and I'm fine," she says [1].

As you move forward, you're going to have lots and lots of successes. But undoubtedly you're going to have some disappointments, as well. The key is to keep at it.

Here's what you can expect as you take your first steps toward weight loss.

Success ... and Speed Bumps

Jo Ann Hattner, RD, author of Gut Insight and a dietitian in private practice in San Francisco, likes to say, "If you follow it, it works" (a term she says people typically use at Weight Watchers) [2].

Experts say that a healthy weight loss is, on average, about a pound a week, but everyone's body moves at a different pace, so don't get discouraged if your body is a little slower on the uptake [2].

You also probably know that it gets a little harder after you've seen some success. Researchers have studied people who have lost 10 to 20 percent of their body weight in a very controlled setting where food intake and physical activity were measured, says Robert A. Gabbay, MD, PhD, an endocrinologist and director of the Diabetes and Obesity Institute at Pennsylvania State Hershey Medical Center [3].

The result: Their bodies started burning calories less efficiently after the weight loss, which ultimately made the scale start sliding up again even though they hadn't increased the amount of calories they ate or lowered their activity level [3].

"The body makes an adaptation to attempt to force the weight back up," Dr. Gabbay says [3].

What's the solution? People who have gotten over a plateau say they upped their effort. They exercised a little harder and sharpened their focus on getting healthy foods. Once you weigh less, you need to reassess your needs. You may require fewer calories at your new weight [4].

It may also help to lose weight more slowly, Dr. Gabbay says. Your body may fight slow weight loss a little less than it would if you lost ten pounds quickly [3].

Taking baby steps is also a good strategy for motivation. It doesn't matter how much weight you really want to lose, start with very small steps, says Amy Wood, PsyD [5].

"If you try to make too much progress too fast, you'll be quickly overwhelmed and you won't succeed," she says. But with each small step, you'll feel a little better, and you'll be able to take on the next small step and feel even better still, and the process will continue [5].

Take a look at the people who are enrolled in the National Weight Control Registry, a group of people who have lost weight and have been able to keep it off. Some lost weight pretty quickly, but others took as long as fourteen years to get to their goal, but they got there, and they were able to stay there [6].

Another way to outsmart your body's impulse to add the pounds back on is to exercise. Among the people who have enrolled in the National Weight Control Registry, 90 percent say they exercise for about an hour every day, on average [6].

And remember, exercise results in hormone changes that can suppress your appetite, so hunger won't be as much of an issue [7].

Also, don't let the scale get you sidetracked, because it can be terribly fickle. "Your weight can vary two to five pounds in a day, depending on how well hydrated you are or if you had a salty meal the night before," says Kate Hawley, RD [8].

Hattner says she uses her clothes as a guide. "I'm a normal weight for my height, but when I start seeing my clothes getting tight I start recording what I'm eating and looking at my patterns and tightening up on it," she says.

Maintaining a healthy weight is cyclical for everyone. Rather than getting comfy in forgiving sweatpants, do something about a slight weight gain right away, and your weight won't spiral out of control. If you are exercising and eating well the scale may not budge much, but the inches will. You are losing fat and gaining muscle [2]

Pick Yourself Up After a Fall

Along the way, expect to get sidetracked every once in a while. Everybody falls off track once in a while. *Everybody.* And more specifically, you will fall off track every now and again [5].

"You will make mistakes. It's human to be imperfect. The main thing is that you keep trying," Dr. Wood says [5].

The following are some guidelines for picking yourself up when your weight-loss efforts fall through.

Let Go of Negative Thoughts and Get Back on the Plan

"The first step to weight loss is to acknowledge that this is who you are and it's okay," Dr. Wood says. "You may not like your current weight, but you're not going to get anywhere if you beat yourself up" [5].

Rather than spending time criticizing yourself or your body, start creating a vision of who you want to become, then create a strategy and reward yourself for small accomplishments along the way [5].

Lose the "All-or-Nothing" Attitude

If you want to stick to a healthy lifestyle, it's essential to be flexible, Dr. Wood says. When you're too rigid in your expectations of yourself, you'll have the urge to rebel. "Allow yourself to have fun and eat treats now and then," she says [5].

Look for Successes

When you're frustrated by the speed (or lack thereof) of your weight loss, start looking at the other triumphs you've made, Hawley suggests. Maybe it's time to get your lipid or glucose levels checked to see if there's been an improvement, she says. Or notice how much easier it is to climb a set of stairs. Or look at your exercise log, and calculate how many miles you've biked, walked, or run since starting your weight-loss journey [8].

Focus on What You Can Have, Rather Than What You Can't

People tend to fixate on what they shouldn't eat when they're trying to lose weight, Gans says. We live in a world where nobody likes to be deprived, but having that type of deprivation-oriented thinking can cause cravings, which can get you off track. Let go of the idea of eating the impossibly big ice cream sundae and start drooling over the healthy berry crisp you can make instead. Think about all the new types of foods you can try such as quinoa, and experiment with new fruits and vegetables. Dragonfruit anyone? [1]

Lean on a Friend

When you surround yourself with people and put yourself in situations that make you feel good about yourself, you're more likely to be able to stick it out after a slip, Dr. Wood says. What not to do: Keep toxic friends in your life. The negativity will drain the energy you need to act on healthful decisions [5].

Purge the Clutter

Just as you don't want to spend time with people who aren't supporting you, you shouldn't keep life "clutter" that may be holding you back. That goes for all of the stuff that may be cluttering your space, obligations, goals, and ideas that are dragging you down, Dr. Wood says [5].

"They're taking up premium space," Dr. Wood says. "When you release what's not serving you positively, you will create space for new and better opportunities that encourage your healthful living goals" [5].

Appreciate Your Body's Own Timeline

"People say to me, 'I've only lost two pounds in the last four months,'" Hattner says. But two pounds is weight loss, she says. You lost two pounds, and you'll lose another two pounds going forward [2].

Have Absolute Faith

You can't succeed otherwise. Establish what you truly have control over, such as the food you bring home and eat out at restaurants, and let the rest go, such as cravings and persuasions from others to eat junk food [5].

"You will find that your intuition and instincts will lead you increasingly to the healthy lifestyle you desire, despite external pressure," Dr. Wood says [5].

Learn Patience for Yourself

You might have patience when it's time to teach your child or grandchild how to ride a bike, but how patient are you with yourself? If you have a setback, it doesn't have to mean it's the end [5].

Weight loss is not easy, but it's doable. Look at all of the successes we've documented in this book through the *What Works for Me* sidebars. There are countless other people out there who are on a journey exactly like the one you're about to embark on.

Every time you make an attempt, you're doing loads of good for your health, Dr. Gabbay says [3].

What Works for Me

Robert Proulx, a retiree living in Dunnellon, FL

As a long-distance cyclist for forty-seven years, I've been fit for most of my life. My family was poor when I was a kid, and getting on my bike and heading out for some free time was my escape. Plus, it didn't cost much to travel by bike.

However, there was a period of time about thirty years ago when I gained ten or fifteen pounds after getting divorced. I was living with my sister and working twelve-hour days at my job. It was also wintertime, so I wasn't able to exercise much. I attribute the weight gain to not being in my own home and working my butt off at my job.

I shed the extra pounds by getting my life back in order, jumping on the bike again for some long rides, eating plenty of fruits and vegetables, and steering clear of processed foods.

(continued)

(continued)

I ride for recreation, but I also use every opportunity I can to hop on my bike. I take my bike to run errands, go out to eat and go shopping, and recently I started riding to my part-time sales job. I average about three thousand miles a year, but this year—with the work commute added—I'm on course to hit about five thousand miles. I do it for my health and to cut down on energy usage.

When I'm not on my bike, I still work on being active by playing tennis, and I've been trying to get more walking in, but I haven't found my motivator for that yet.

Another big factor is the food. I choose to cook my own foods—such as chili and pizza—so I can control what I'm eating. I don't eat beef, chicken, or pork.

I think being in shape is about choosing an activity you enjoy and that fits easily in your everyday lifestyle. It also helps to have friends with whom you can share the activity.

There were times in my past when I considered, but didn't do, more extreme activities, such as riding my bike cross-country, running marathons, and jumping out of airplanes. I've learned that extreme activities cause extreme results, like injuries. Rather than putting a lot of stress on my body trying to push it to its limits, I'd rather choose something that feels good to do every day.

It's a New Day

It's been reported that in the United States we're exposed to three thousand advertisements a day. And let's be honest: Advertisements use perfect bodies to sell products, so we're constantly inundated with pictures of what society tells us is an "ideal" body, even though those images are Photoshopped and airbrushed like crazy [9].

It's true for men and women. Men's bodies on the covers of magazines are beefed up like never before. Women's bodies are perfectly sculpted and, very often, quite thin.

As a result, it's easy to start obsessing about the way your body looks to everyone else, and that type of thinking can lead to low self-esteem and depression, which tend to interfere when you're working on making your lifestyle healthier [9].

Try not to be overly concerned with the number on the scale or your pants size, and know that each step you take today to be healthier is a good thing.

It's good to have healthy goals, but don't let your expectations get out of control. When you have the attitude that you're unhealthy if you're fat and healthy if you're thin, you're creating too much pressure on yourself, Dr. Wood says. Your thinking might go in a negative direction, like this: "The only way I can be healthy is to lose all this weight, and since I can't do it now, why try?" [5]

Another thing: Start loving the way you look right now—before losing a single pound [5]. Ladies, go out and buy some up-to-date clothes. (Check out some online fashion blogs—from women of all sizes—if you're not sure what to buy.) Go out and get a manicure or some makeup.

Men, add some dashing pieces to your wardrobe or get a good haircut and a refreshing shave.

While you're at it, you might as well get some workout clothes that will make you feel good while you exercise.

When you start dressing and acting like the healthier person you want to be, you'll make more and more decisions in line with what that healthier person needs—that may mean pushing your chair away from the dinner table after you've had enough, going out for a run even when you're feeling lazy, or passing up an invitation to eat lunch at a fast-food joint for the wrap you stashed in your lunch bag [5].

The beast—hunger—will rule no longer.

Take Dr. Wood's advice: Make the art of living well a daily practice. "Look at each day as a new day and a fresh opportunity to treat yourself well," she says [5].

Before you know it, voilà, the new you will be here [5].

TEN RULES TO LIVE BY:

1. Honor your hunger.
2. Stay in touch with your satiety.
3. Eat satisfying meals and snacks.
4. Record everything you eat in a food journal.
5. Be prepared with the tools you need.
6. Keep moving your body.
7. Take small steps toward your goal.
8. Show your body respect.
9. Know that you can lose weight.
10. Celebrate every success, no matter how big or small.

Dietitian's Diary

We're With You as You Move On

As you embark on your new journey, you will learn more about yourself and life-changing, sustainable weight loss. It may be one of the most difficult things you've ever done. But you can do it! And you can keep that weight off! We have not just shown you a gimmick or a quick fix. It took time to gain weight, and it will take time to lose it.

At first, change is hard. Talk to anyone in recovery from an addiction. But just keep moving. Every day will get better. Every day is part of the learning and growing process. You will learn more about your strengths and weaknesses as you meet your goals. Just remember, there will be times when you will come up short. At times you will struggle with motivating yourself to exercise, choosing healthier foods, dealing with stress without food, and making sure to get enough healing sleep. But it will get easier as you learn about how you are affected by certain situations. For instance, I really enjoy wine and cheese. Both are calorie laden and definitely not healthy in large quantities at one sitting. So, my goal is to cut off 1 to 2 ounces of cheese and pour one glass of wine. Then, I put it away or walk away from the buffet table. My weakness is wine and cheese. My strength is my ability to enjoy every last sip of wine and nibble of cheese.

Food is not just nourishment; it is life. It is emotional, it is social, and, for some, it has been scary. Stop letting food and your body hold you back from real health. Lose weight one day at a time through good decisions, and you can add more years to your life. If you don't believe you can by now, then dig deep. It's never too late for anyone to change his/her life. You may feel like you never follow through with anything, but let me remind you that you are just about to finish reading a book that you can let change your life.

Keep positive. Only you can make or break your accomplishment in health. So, immerse yourself in positive thought, and surround yourself with encouraging people. Allow yourself to let go of fear and loathing of whatever it is that might hold you back. What is your motivation for being a healthier weight? Is it to run around with your kids now, or is it to watch your grandchildren grow up? Is it to not break a sweat while going up a flight of stairs? Or is it the excitement of being able to purchase a hot pair of jeans several sizes smaller than the ones in your closet? Whatever your reason, hold onto it. Whatever it is, the feeling it brings will last longer than the taste of comfort food.

Besides life and health goals, ask yourself what externally motivates you. What type of music will push you that extra minute on the treadmill? How will you treat yourself after achieving your food goals throughout the week? Do you have a favorite quote to recite for motivation? I like to take a dry-erase marker to my bathroom mirror and write a positive quote or Bible verse. Here is what is on my mirror right now:

> **"Nothing in the world is worth having or worth doing unless it means effort, pain, and difficulty."**
>
> **President Theodore Roosevelt**

You are going to feel better than you ever thought you could. But remember, it will not happen overnight. It will happen after many exhausting workouts, delicious satisfying meals, and restful nights of sleep. And in the end, it will all be worth it!

More Recipes for Your New, Healthy Life

(Arranged alphabetically)

ASIAN CUCUMBER SALAD   Serves: 4

1 teaspoon sea salt
⅛ cup sesame seeds, toasted
1 English cucumber, sliced

½ teaspoon fresh ground black pepper
1 tablespoon sesame oil, toasted
2 tablespoons soy sauce, low sodium
1 tablespoon garlic, minced
1 tablespoon sugar
¼ cup water
¾ cup rice vinegar, seasoned

Directions:

1. Combine all ingredients together.

2. Serve cold.

Per serving: 83 calories, 3.75 g fat, 11 g carbohydrate, 0.4 g fiber, 1.3 g protein.

ASIAN FLANK STEAK   Serves: 6

12 ounces flank steak
⅛ cup soy sauce, low sodium
3 tablespoons brown sugar
1 tablespoon garlic, minced
3 tablespoons sesame oil, toasted
1 tablespoon rice vinegar, seasoned
1 tablespoon olive oil, extra virgin
1 tablespoon Chinese 5-spice powder
½ tablespoon ginger root, grated
2 green onions, diced

Directions:

1. Combine all ingredients in a bowl (except steak).

2. Put ⅛ cup of sauce in a separate bowl (the rest will be used for dipping sauce to serve).

3. Using a nonstick pan or the grill, cook steak.

4. When steak has about 5 minutes left to cook, brush with sauce from ⅛ cup that was set aside.

5. Let meat rest for about 5 minutes off of heat.

6. Serve with dipping sauce.

Per serving: 190 calories, 13 g fat, 6 g carbohydrate, 0.1 g fiber, 12.3 g protein.

BAKED OATMEAL GRANOLA CASSEROLE   **Serves: 10**

Cooking spray, to coat pan for baking
1 pint blueberries, fresh
2 apples, cored and diced
1½ cups soy milk
1 teaspoon vanilla extract
1 teaspoon cinnamon
½ teaspoon coarse salt
2 teaspoons baking powder
3 egg whites
½ cup brown sugar
4 cups oatmeal, old fashioned
¼ cup canola oil
1 cup fruit, dried, mixed

Directions:

1. Preheat oven to 350 degrees.

2. Combine all ingredients in a bowl.

3. Mix through.

4. Spray a baking pan to coat.

5. Add oatmeal mixtures to pan.

6. Cook for 30 minutes, or until a light golden brown.

Per serving 307 calories, 8.2 g fat, 50.5 g carbohydrate, 2.3 g fiber, 7.8 g protein.

BLACK-EYED PEA SALAD   **Serves: 8**

3 cups black-eyed peas, frozen
2 tomatoes, chopped
½ cup yellow onion, diced
½ cup cilantro, fresh, chopped

Dressing:

½ tablespoon chili powder,
2 tablespoons garlic, minced

⅛ cup apple cider vinegar
1 tablespoon olive oil, extra virgin
1 tablespoon honey
1 lemon juice, fresh

Directions:

1. Cook black-eyed peas according to package.

2. While peas are cooking, prepare remaining ingredients for salad.

3. Prepare dressing by stirring together the above ingredients.

4. When peas are done cooking, drain off the cooking water.

5. Cool peas to room temperature by rinsing with cool water.

6. In serving dish, combine the remaining ingredients for salad.

7. Add dressing to your desired taste.

8. Serve cold.

Per Serving: 130 calories, 2.3 g fat, 21.3 g carbohydrate, 1.4 g fiber, 6.1 g protein

BREAKFAST SMOOTHIE   **Serves: 2**

½ 12 oz. package(s) tofu, silken
1 cup strawberries, unsweetened, frozen
½ cup orange juice, fortified with vitamin D and calcium
1 cup kale, chopped, frozen
1 apple, cored and chopped (leave skin on)
1 tablespoon flaxseed meal

Directions:

1. Drain excess water from tofu.

2. Combine all ingredients in a food processor or blender.

3. Add extra water or orange juice if a more liquid consistence is desired.

Per serving: 229 calories, 5.6 g fat, 34.4 g carbohydrate, 3.9 g fiber, 10.2 g protein.

CHOCOLATE-COVERED CHERRY QUINOA PORRIDGE   Serves: 4

1 cup quinoa, flakes
1½ cups chocolate soy milk
3 teaspoons caramel extract
8 tablespoons dried cherries

Directions:

1. Cook quinoa according to package directions with the chocolate soy milk as the liquid.

2. Stir in extract and dried cherries.

3. Enjoy warm.

TIP
Make several batches at a time. Freeze some and thaw in the refrigerator for later use.

Per serving: 200 calories, 2 g fat, 39.6 g carbohydrate, 3.1 g fiber, 5.6 g protein.

CILANTRO SAUCE   Serves: 6

1 medium lime rind
2 tablespoons garlic, minced
2 cups cilantro (about one bunch)
2 tablespoons pineapple preserves
½ tablespoon red chili paste
2 tablespoons sweet chili sauce
2 tablespoons soy sauce, low sodium
Juice from one medium lime

Directions:

1. Puree all of the above in a food processor or blender.

2. Use a dipping sauce or a barbequing sauce for chicken or pork.

Per serving: 34 calories, 0 g fat, 7.4 g carbohydrate, 0.3 g fiber, 1 g protein.

COLORFUL PASTA WITH VEGETABLES   Serves: 6

1 box multicolored spiral pasta, whole grain (12 oz)
1 bunch broccoli
1 head cauliflower
½ cup walnuts
3 tablespoons olive oil
2 tablespoons garlic, minced
¼ cup grated parmesan cheese
1 tablespoon butter
Pepper to taste

Directions:

1. Cook pasta.
2. While pasta is cooking, boil more water for the vegetables.
3. Trim cauliflower and broccoli to cook just the florets.
4. Blanch vegetables in boiling water.
5. Drain water from the vegetables pot. Set vegetables aside in another bowl.
6. Heat olive oil in pot and sauté garlic. When garlic is almost transparent add in walnuts.
7. Lightly toast walnuts.
8. Add vegetables back to pot and warm through. Turn off stove.
9. Drain pasta and add to vegetable mixture.
10. Stir in butter and cheese to melt.

Season to taste with pepper.
Per serving: 439 calories, 18 g fat, 53 g carbohydrate, 3.7 g fiber, 16 g protein.

FENNEL WITH CANNELLINI BEANS   Serves: 8

2 tablespoons olive oil
2 tablespoons white balsamic vinegar
1 teaspoon dried thyme
¼ teaspoon pepper
3 fennel bulbs
2 cans cannellini beans, drained and rinsed

Directions:

1. In a large bowl mix together oil, vinegar, and seasonings.

2. Trim off green stalks from fennel.

3. Chop fennel into desired bite-size pieces, or slice with food processor for an even cut.

4. Toss beans and fennel with dressing.

5. Serve chilled.

Per serving: 112 calories, 3.5 g fat, 14 g carbohydrate, 0.6 g fiber, 6 g protein.

GREEK SALAD   Serves: 10

12 medium Kalamata olives, sliced
½ cup olive juice, from olive jar
½ cup red onion, diced
1 tablespoon olive oil, extra virgin
2 medium tomatoes, chopped
1 large English cucumber, chopped
1 medium green bell pepper, diced
1 cup Italian parsley, lightly packed, chopped
2 tablespoons oregano, dried
2 cups brown rice, cooked and chilled

Directions:

1. Combine all in a serving bowl.

2. Serve cold.

Per serving: 179 calories, 4 g fat, 32 g carbohydrate, 1 g fiber, 3.5 g protein.

HEARTS OF PALM SALAD   Serves: 4

1 14 oz. can hearts of palm, drained and chopped
1 medium tomato, chopped
1 medium avocado, cubed
2 tablespoons olive oil, extra virgin
1 tablespoon orange juice
1 tablespoon lime juice
Sea salt and fresh ground pepper, to taste

Directions:

1. Combine all in a bowl.
2. Serve cold.

TIP

For extra satisfaction, serve with salad greens.

Per serving: 183 calories, 14.5 g fat, 9.1 g carbohydrate, 2.4 g fiber, 3.9 g protein.

PARSLEY PESTO   Serves: 12

1 cup Italian parsley
½ cup basil leaves, fresh
1 tablespoon parmesan cheese
⅛ cup water
¼ cup walnuts
½ tablespoon lemon juice, fresh
1 tablespoon garlic, diced
2 tablespoons olive oil, extra virgin

Directions:

1. Combine all ingredients in a food processor or blender.
2. Puree until smooth.

TIPS

1. Use fresh parmesan cheese from the deli for excellent flavor.
2. Make more than one recipe and freeze some for later. Thaw in the fridge and serve.

Per serving: 44 calories, 3.9 g fat, 1.5 g carbohydrate, 0.3 g fiber, 0.8 g protein.

PINEAPPLE PORK LOIN AND SWEET PARSNIPS   Serves: 5

4 parsnips, thinly sliced
2 cups quinoa, red
4 tablespoons pineapple preserves
2 cups vegetable broth
3 tablespoons mint leaves, fresh
4 tablespoons white wine vinegar
10 oz. pork loin

Directions:

1. Cook red quinoa according to package.
2. Boil water and add parsnips. Cook until soft, or steam instead if desired.
3. Wash pork loin and evenly spread preserves on loin.
4. Heat a nonstick pan and lightly coat with nonstick spray.
5. Sear non-preserve side of pork for 2 minutes on medium-low heat.
6. Turn pork over with preserve side down. Turn heat to low.
7. Cook for 3 minutes on low.
8. Add vegetable broth to pan and cover.
9. Cook on low for about 10 minutes or until cooked to preference.
10. Remove pork from pan and set aside to keep warm.
11. Add mint and vinegar to pan.
12. Deglaze pan to create a sweet sauce.
13. Serve vegetables atop quinoa and 2 ounces of meat on the side. Top with sauce.

TIPS
1. Place the pork on a plate and set in microwave to keep warm.
2. Cook extra pork for another meal, such as Fajita Pasta.

Per serving: 413 calories, 7 g fat, 62 g carbohydrate, 4.5 g fiber, 24.6 g protein.

RED STRAWBLUBERRY QUINOA   **Serves: 5**

1 cup red quinoa
1½ cups nonfat milk
3 teaspoons strawberry extract
8 tablespoons dried blueberries

Directions:

1. Combine 1½ cups of nonfat milk and 1 cup rinsed quinoa.

2. Bring to a boil.

3. Turn down heat and simmer for 15 minutes.

4. Remove from heat.

5. Let sit 5 minutes.

6. Stir in strawberry extract and dried blueberries.

Per serving: 326 calories, 16.2 g fat, 37.2 g carbohydrate, 5.7 g fiber, 7.7 g protein

SATISFACTION SOLUTION OATMEAL   **Serves: 2**

1 cup oats, quick cooking
1 ounce pecan halves
2 tablespoons flaxseed meal
2 teaspoons rum extract

Directions:

1. Cook oatmeal according to package with water as the liquid.

2. Stir in remaining ingredients and enjoy warm.

TIP
Store extra in the refrigerator and reheat for the next day for breakfast or a sweet snack.

Per serving: 282 calories, 13.3 g fat, 32.3 g carbohydrate, 2.5 g fiber, 8.3 g protein.

SATISFACTION SOLUTION WRAP   **Serves: 1**

1 FlatOut multigrain wrap
1 ounce provolone cheese
½ cup spinach
⅛ cup red bell pepper
⅛ cup jicama
⅛ cup carrot, diced
⅛ cup corn kernels, frozen
1 tablespoon mayonnaise, canola or vegenaise
2 tablespoons cilantro, chopped

Directions:

1. Rinse corn in room-temperature water to slightly thaw and remove frost.

2. Combine all ingredients (except cheese) into a bowl and mix through.

3. Place cheese and vegetables onto wrap.

4. Wrap up the mixture and enjoy!

TIP

If you bring your wrap to school or work for lunch, pack the vegetable mixture separate from the wrap and assemble when time to eat. This will help prevent a soggy wrap.

Per serving: 368 calories, 20.9 g fat, 27 g carbohydrate, 8.8 g fiber, 18 g protein.

SIMPLE PASTA SAUCE   **Serves: 6**

2 15 oz. cans tomatoes, diced
2 medium green bell peppers, chopped
1 cup yellow onion, chopped
1 cup red onion, chopped
2 cups fresh basil, chopped
2 tablespoons garlic, minced
2 tablespoons oregano, dried
2 tablespoons balsamic vinegar

1 tablespoon sea salt
2 tablespoons olive oil, extra virgin

Directions:

1. Sautee peppers, onion, and garlic in olive oil until yellow onion is translucent.

2. Add remaining ingredients.

3. Simmer for 25 minutes.

TIP
Make extra and freeze for later. Thaw in the refrigerator.

Per serving: 129 calories, 5 g fat, 18 g carbohydrate, 2.5 g fiber, 3 g protein.

SOUTHWEST CORN AVOCADO DIP   Serves: 8

2 avocados, mashed
1 cup white beans, mashed
1 tablespoon liquid smoke
1 juice of lime
¼ teaspoon chili powder
2 plum tomatoes, chopped
3 green onions, chopped
¼ cup cilantro, chopped
1 cup corn kernels, frozen
Sea salt, to taste

Directions:

1. Mash avocado and white beans together.

2. Stir in seasonings (liquid smoke, lime juice, and chili powder).

3. Rinse frozen corn in room temperature water to slightly thaw and remove frost.

4. Gently fold in remaining ingredients (tomatoes, green onion, corn, and cilantro).

Per serving: 154 calories, 8.1 g fat, 16.4 g carbohydrate, 2 g fiber, 3.9 g protein.

SPICY MANGO CILANTRO SOUP   **Serves: 4**

3 mangoes, peeled and pitted
2 tablespoons honey
2 juice of two limes
½ teaspoon chili powder
1 teaspoon cumin
1 cup cilantro

Directions:

1. Put all ingredients in blender or food processor.

2. Serve cold.

Per serving: 150 calories, 0.6 g fat, 35.1 g carbohydrate, 1.4 g fiber, 1 g protein.

SWEET MEXICAN SALAD   **Serves: 4**

1 15 oz. can black beans, drained and rinsed
1 medium mango, pitted and diced
½ cup jicama, diced
½ cup cilantro, loosely packed, chopped
1 medium lime, juice and zest
1 medium Bosc pear, chopped
1 tablespoon white balsamic vinegar

Directions:

1. Combine together in a serving dish.

2. Serve chilled as is or on top of salad greens for additional satisfaction.

Per serving: 220 calories, 0.9 g fat, 42.8 g carbohydrate, 3.3 g fiber, 10.1 g protein.

TOFU VEGETABLE DIP   **Serves: 4**

½ 12 oz. tofu, silken (half of a package)
3 tablespoons Mrs. Dash Italian Blend
1 tablespoon Mrs. Dash Garlic and Herb Blend

Directions:

1. Mix all ingredients together to combine until smooth.

2. Serve chilled.

TIP

Use tofu for dips instead of sour cream. You save on calories and get healthy phytochemicals and protein from the tofu.

Per serving: 41 calories, 2 g fat, 2.2 g carbohydrate, 0 g fiber, 3.4 g protein.

TORTILLA SALAD   Serves: 10

1 16 oz. package corn kernels, frozen
1 15 oz. can black beans, canned, drained and rinsed
2 red bell peppers, chopped
1 cup red onion, diced
¼ cup cilantro, fresh, chopped
½ cup salsa
1 avocado, diced
3 cups romaine lettuce

Directions:

1. Rinse frozen corn in a colander with room-temperature water from about 45 seconds to remove frost.

2. Combine black beans through avocado in a serving bowl and stir gently.

3. Serve atop romaine lettuce.

Per serving: 152 calories, 3.6 g fat, 24 g carbohydrate, 2 g fiber, 6 g protein.

WATERMELON SALAD   Serves: 6

4 cups watermelon, chopped
2 green onions, diced

Dressing:

1½ juice of (one and a half) limes
1½ zest of (one and a half) limes
2 tablespoons honey
3 tablespoons cilantro, fresh, chopped
½ teaspoon chili powder

1 teaspoon sea salt
½ teaspoon ginger root, grated

Directions:

1. Combine ingredients of dressing. Mix well.
2. In serving bowl, combine onion and watermelon.
3. Gently combine dressing and watermelon mixture.
4. Serve cold.

Per serving: 62 calories, 0.5 g fat, 13.6 g carbohydrate, 0.4 g fiber, 0.8 g protein.

WHITE BEANS WITH PARSLEY PESTO   Serves: 6

1 15 oz. can cannellini beans, drained and rinsed
2 medium tomatoes, chopped
½ cup red onion, diced
Half a recipe of Parsley Pesto (Page 247)

Directions:

1. Combine all ingredients together and mix well.
2. Serve chilled.

Per serving: 71.6 calories, 0.6 g fat, 12 g carbohydrate, 0.6 g fiber, 4.5 g protein.

References

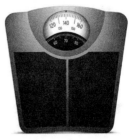

Chapter 1

1. Interview with Richard J. Lindquist, MD, Medical program director and a bariatric physician, Swedish Weight Loss Services, Seattle, WA.
2. National Diabetes Information Clearinghouse. "Insulin Resistance and Pre-diabetes." http://diabetes.niddk.nih.gov/dm/pubs/insulinresistance/.
3. Druce M. R., A. M. Wren, A. J. Park, J. E. Milton, M. Patterson, G. Frost, M. A. Ghatei, C. Small, and S. R. Bloom. September 2005. "Ghrelin Increases Food Intake in Obese as Well as Lean Subjects." *International Journal of Obesity* 29 (9): 1130–6. Accessed June 2011. http://www.ncbi.nlm.nih.gov/pubmed/15917842.
4. "Action of Ghrelin Hormone Increases Appetite and Favor Accumulation of Abdominal Fat." *ScienceDaily.* Accessed June 2011. http://www.sciencedaily.com/releases/2009/05/090520055519.htm.
5. Klok, M. D., S. Jakobsdottir, and M. L. Drent. January 2007. "The Role of Leptin and Ghrelin in the Regulation of Food Intake and Body Weight in Humans: A Review." *Obesity Reviews* 8 (1): 21–24. Accessed June 2011. http://onlinelibrary.wiley.com/doi/10.1111/j.1467-789X.2006.00270.x/full.
6. Paddon-Jones, D., E. Westman, R. D. Mattes, R. R. Wolfe, A. Astrup, and M. Westerterp-Plantenga. May 2008. "Protein, Weight Management, and Satiety." *American Journal of Clinical Nutrition* 87 (5): 1558S–1561S. Accessed June 2011. http://www.ajcn.org/content/87/5/1558S.full.
7. Ciampolini, M., D. Lovell-Smith, R. Bianchi, B. de Pont, M. Sifone, M. van Weeren, W. de Hahn, L. Borselli, and A. Pietrobelli. 2010.

"Sustained Self-Regulation of Energy Intake: Initial Hunger Improves Insulin Sensitivity." *Journal of Nutrition and Metabolism* 2010, Article ID 286952. http://www.hindawi.com/journals/jnume/2010/286952/

8. Harvard Health Publications. "Abdominal Fat and What to Do About It." http://www.health.harvard.edu/newsweek/Abdominal-fat-and-what-to-do-about-it.htm.

9. Teff, Karen L., S. S. Elliott, M. Tschöp, T. J. Kieffer, D. Rader, M. Heiman, R. R. Townsend, N. L. Keim, D. D'Alessio, and P. J. Havel. 2004. "Dietary Fructose Reduces Circulating Insulin and Leptin, Attenuates Postpradial Suppression of Ghrelin and Increases Triglycerides in Women." *Journal of Clinical Endocrinology and Metabolism* 89 (6). http://jcem.endojournals.org/cgi/content/abstract/89/6/2963.

10. Interview with Dana Simpler, MD, a physician at Mercy Medical Center, Baltimore, MD.

11. Mayo Clinic. "Digestion: How Long Does it Take?" http://www.mayoclinic.com/health/digestive-system/an00896.

12. Yale Medical Group. "Weight-Loss Surgery has Benefits Beyond Slimming Down." http://www.yalemedicalgroup.org/bell_12282009.

13. Interview with Patience White, MD, chief public health officer of the Arthritis Foundation, adult and pediatric rheumatologist, and a professor of medicine and pediatrics, George Washington University.

14. American Diabetes Association. "Healthy Weight Loss." http://www.diabetes.org/food-and-fitness/fitness/weight-loss/healthy-weight-loss.html.

15. Centers for Disease Control and Prevention. "Losing Weight." http://www.cdc.gov/healthyweight/losing_weight/index.html.

16. Inova Health System. "Benefits of Weight Loss." http://www.inova.org/healthcare-services/weight-loss/benefits-of-weight-loss.

17. Weight Watchers. "Unexpected Benefits of Weight Loss." http://www.weightwatchers.com/util/art/index_art.aspx?tabnum=1&art_id=34381&sc=3047.

18. "Sex and Weight." *Psychology Today*. http://www.psychologytoday.com/blog/all-about-sex/201005/sex-and-weight.

Chapter 2

1. Interview with Theresa Piotrowski, MD, Medical director of the Medical and Surgical Weight Loss Center, The Lahey Clinic, Boston.

2. Interview with Christy D. Hofsess, PhD, Licensed psychologist and assistant professor, Department of Counseling and Health Psychology, Bastyr University, Kenmore, WA.

3. Harvard School of Public Health. "The Nutrition Source: Food Pyramids: What Should You Really Eat?" http://www.hsph.harvard.edu/nutrition-source/what-should-you-eat/pyramid-full-story/index.html.

4. "BMI and Calorie Calculator." USDA/ARS Children's Nutrition Research Center at Baylor College of Medicine. http://www.bcm.edu/cnrc/caloriesneed.htm.

5. "Daily Food Plan." U.S. Department of Agriculture, MyPyramid, http://www.mypyramid.gov/mypyramid/index.aspx.

6. Interview with Keri Gans, RD, Author of The Small-Change Diet, nutritionist in private practice, New York City.

7. Interview with Barbara Mendez, Nutritionist and registered pharmacist and owner of Barbara Mendez Nutrition, barbara@lifestylenutrients.net.

8. National Eating Disorders Association. "Factors That May Contribute to Eating Disorders." http://www.nationaleatingdisorders.org/uploads/file/information-resources/Factors%20that%20may%20Contribute%20to%20Eating%20Disorders.pdf.

9. U.S. Department of Health and Human Services. "Binge Eating Disorder, The National Women's Health Information Center." http://www.womenshealth.gov/faq/binge-eating-disorder.cfm.

10. Interview with Amy Wood, PsyD, A psychologist in private practice, in Portland, Maine, and author of Life Your Way. amywood@amywoodpsyd.com.

11. "Food Cravings, Types of Cravings, and Weight Management." July 19, 2007. ScienceDaily. Accessed June 2011. http://www.sciencedaily.com/releases/2007/07/070718001508.htm.

12. "The Psychology of Food Cravings." May 18, 2010. ScienceDaily, Accessed June 2011. http://www.sciencedaily.com/releases/2010/05/100517172300.htm.

13. Interview with Richard J. Lindquist, MD, Medical program director and a bariatric physician, Swedish Weight Loss Services, Seattle, WA.

14. Taylor, A. H., and A. J. Oliver. February 2009. "Effect of Brisk Walking on Urges to Eat Chocolate, Affect, and Responses to a Stressor and Chocolate Cue. An Experimental Study." Appetite 52 (1). Accessed June 2011. http://www.ncbi.nlm.nih.gov/pubmed/18835411.

15. Taubert, D., R. Roesen, C. Lehmann, N. Jung, and E. Schömig. July 4, 2007. "Effects of Low Habitual Cocoa Intake on Blood Pressure and

Bioactive Nitric Oxide." 2007. *Journal of the American Medical Association.* 298 (1). http://jama.ama-assn.org/content/298/1/49.full.

16. Chen, L., L. J. Appel, C. Loria, P. H. Lin, C. M. Champagne, P. J. Elmer, J. D. Ard, et al. May 2009. "Reduction in the Consumption of Sugar-Sweetened Beverages Is Associated with Weight Loss: The Premier Trial." *American Journal of Clinical Nutrition* 89 (5): 1299–1306. Accessed June 2011. http://www.ajcn.org/content/89/5/1299.full?sid=992f2076-406a-4978-ad63-ffce65ec9841.

17. Lipton's Iced Teas: Lipton Brisk, Raspberry, http://www.calorieking.com/foods/calories-in-iced-teas-lipton-brisk-raspberry_f-ZmlkPTc0NzE3.html.

18. Swithers, Susan E., and Terry L. Davidson. February 2008. "A Role for Sweet Taste: Calorie Predictive Relations in Energy Regulation by Rats." *Behavioral Neuroscience* 122 (1): 161–173. Accessed June 2011. http://psycnet.apa.org/journals/bne/122/1/161/

19. http://dailyburn.com/nutrition/cargill_truvia_calories.

20. Davis, E. 1995. "Functionality of Sugars: Physicochemical Interactions in Foods," *American Journal of Clinical Nutrition* 62 (suppl.): 170S–77S.

21. Cummings, J. H., G. T. Macfarlane, and H. N. Englyst. 2001. "Prebiotic Digestion and Fermentation." *American Journal of Clinical Nutrition* 73 (2 Suppl): 415S–20S.

22. Drewnowski, A. 1999. "Sweetness, Appetite, and Energy Intake: Physiological Aspects." *World Review, Nutrition and Dietetics* 85: 64–76. Basel, Switzerland: S. Karger AG.

23. Drewnowski, A. 1995. "Intense Sweeteners and the Control of Appetite." *Nutrition Review* 53: 1–7.

24. Duffy, V., and M. Sigman-Grant. 2004. "Position of the American Dietetic Association: Use of Nutritive and Nonnutritive Sweeteners." *Journal of the American Dietetic Association* 104: 255–75.

Chapter 3

1. Interview with Jackie Newgent, RD, culinary nutritionist and author of *Big Green Cookbook: Hundreds of Planet-Pleasing Recipes & Tips for a Luscious, Low-Carbon Lifestyle*, New York City.

2. Interview with Christy D. Hofsess, PhD, Licensed psychologist and assistant professor in the Department of Counseling and Health Psychology, Bastyr University, Kenmore, WA, chofsess@bastyr.edu.

3. Partnership for Essential Nutrition. "The Impact of the Low-Carb Craze on Attitudes About Eating and Weight Loss." http://www.essentialnutrition. org/survey.php.

4. University of Illinois at Urbana-Champaign. "Essentials for Eaters and Dieters: Healthy Lifestyles." http://efed.aces.uiuc.edu/101/healthyeat. html.

5. Interview with Amy Wood, PsyD, a psychologist in private practice, in Portland, Maine, and author of *Life Your Way*.

6. Center for Mindful Eating. "The Principles of Mindful Eating." http:// www.tcme.org/principles.htm.

7. Interview with H. Theresa Wright, RD, founder of Renaissance Nutrition Center, Inc., East Norriton, PA.

8. CalorieKing.com.

9. Pop chips: http://www.popchips.com/nutrition-information/

10. Centers for Disease Control and Prevention. "Do Increased Portion Sizes Affect how Much We Eat?" http://www.tcme.org/principles.htm.

11. Family Doctor. "Fad Diets." http://familydoctor.org/online/famdocen/ home/healthy/food/improve/784.html.

12. Interview with Naomi Lippel, managing director of Overeaters Anonymous, Inc., Rio Rancho, NM.

13. "Basic Information about the OA Fellowship." *Overeaters Anonymous*, http:// www.oa.org/media-resources/

Chapter 4

1. Calorie Control Council Lighten Up and Get Moving activity calculator, http://www.caloriecontrol.org/healthy-weight-tool-kit/lighten-up-and-get-moving.

2. Interview with Shaun A. Zetlin, a certified master trainer in the New York metro area, certified through the National Academy of Sports Medicine as a personal trainer and certified by the International Sports Science Association as a Sport Performance Nutrition Specialist, info@ zetlinfitness.com, www.zetlinfitness.com.

3. Broom, David R., R. L. Batterham, J. A. King, and D. J. Stensel. January 2009. "Influence of Resistance and Aerobic Exercise on hunger, Circulating Levels of Acylated ghrelin, and Peptide YY in Healthy Males." *American Journal of Physiology* 296 (1). Accessed March 2011. http://ajpregu.physiology.org/ content/296/1/R29.full.

4. "Exercise Suppresses Appetite by Affecting Appetite Hormones." December 19, 2008. *ScienceDaily*, Accessed March 2011. http://www. sciencedaily.com/releases/2008/12/081211081446.htm.

5. Interview with Christina Walman, a group fitness instructor for twenty years, Santa Barbara, CA. christina.walman@changeleader.com.

6. National Weight Control Registry. "NWCR Facts." http://www.nwcr.ws/ Research/default.htm.

7. "Exercise Alone Shown to Improve Insulin Sensitivity in Obese Sedentary Adolescents." September 11, 2009. *ScienceDaily*, Accessed March 2011. http://www.sciencedaily.com/releases/2009/09/090901082406.htm.

8. Puetz, Timothy W., S. S. Flowers, and P. J. O'Connor. March 2008. "A Randomized Controlled Trial of the Effect of Aerobic Exercise Training on Feelings of Energy and Fatigue in Sedentary Young Adults with Persistent Fatigue." *Psychotherapy and Psychosomatics* 77 (3). Accessed March 2011. http://content.karger.com/produktedb/produkte. asp?DOI=10.1159/000116610.

9. "Low-Intensity Exercise Reduces Fatigue Symptoms by 65 Percent, Study Finds." *ScienceDaily*, March 2, 2008. http://www.sciencedaily.com/ releases/2008/02/080228112008.htm.

10. Smits, Jasper, and Michael, Otto 2009. *Exercise for Mood and Anxiety Disorders: Therapist Guide (Treatments That Work)*. Amazon listing and news articles. http://psychcentral.com/news/2010/04/06/exercise-ther-apy-for-depression/12627.html, http://www.sciencedaily.com/ releases/2010/04/100405122311.htm, http://www usatoday. com/news/health/painter/2010-04-26-yourhealth26_ST_N.htm, http://www.amazon.com/gp/product/0195382250/ref=pd_lpo_ k2_dp_sr_2?pf_rd_p=486539851&pf_rd_s=lpo-top-stripe-1&pf_ rd_t=201&pf_rd_i=0195382269&pf_rd_m=ATVPDKIKX0DER& pf_rd_r=1RYHNDSZS43Z2BPCNDF9.

11. Crystal Petrello.

12. Jakicic, John M., B .H .Marcus, W. Lang, and C. Janney. July 2008. "Effect of Exercise on 24-Month Weight Loss Maintenance in Overweight Women." *Archives of Internal Medicine* 168 (14). Accessed March 2011. http://archinte. ama-assn.org/cgi/content/full/168/14/1550.

13. Schmidt, W. D, C. J. Biwer, and L. K. Kalscheuer. October 2001. "Effects of Long versus Short Bouts of Exercise on Fitness and Weight Loss in Over-weight Females." Journal of the American College of Nutrition 20 (5). http://www.jacn.org/content/20/5/494.full

14. ACE exercise library: http://www.acefitness.org/exerciselibrary/default. aspx.

Chapter 5

1. U.S. Department of Agriculture. "Safe Food Handling: Freezing and Food Safety." http://www.fsis.usda.gov/factsheets/focus_on_freezing/index.asp.
2. Interview with Melissa Paris, Certified nutritionist, certified personal trainer, and owner of Melissa Paris Fitness, New York City.
3. "Menu Labeling in Chain Restaurants. Opportunities for Public Policy." 2008. *Rudd Report*, Rudd Center for Food Policy and Obesity at Yale University, http://www.yaleruddcenter.org/resources/upload/docs/what/reports/RuddMenuLabelingReport2008.pdf.
4. Center for Science and the Public Interest. "Nutrition Labeling at Fast-Food and Other Chain Restaurants." http://www.cspinet.org/menulabeling/why.pdf.
5. Center for Science in the Public Interest. July 19, 2011. "Eating is as Xtreme as Ever in America's Chain." Accessed August 2011. http://www.cspinet.org/new/201107191.html.
6. Interview with Robert A. Gabbay, MD, PhD, An endocrinologist at Pennsylvania State Hershey Medical Center, director of Penn State Hershey Diabetes and Obesity Institute, Hersehy, PA.
7. Dunkin' Donuts website. https://www.dunkindonuts.com
8. Starbucks website. http://www.starbucks.com/
9. Burger King website. http://www.bk.com/
10. McDonald's website. http://www.mcdonalds.com
11. CalorieKing.com. http://www.calorieking.com/
12. Cosi website. http://www.getcosi.com/
13. On the Border website. http://www.ontheborder.com/
14. Macaroni Grill website. http://www.macaronigrill.com/
15. Outback Steakhouse website. http://www.outback.com/
16. Olive Garden website. http://www.olivegarden.com/
17. Interview with H. Theresa Wright, MS, RD, LDN, Founder of Renaissance Nutrition Center.

Chapter 6

1. Leahey, T. M., J. Gokee LaRose, J. L. Fava, and R. R. Wing. June 2011. "Social Influences Are Associated with BMI and Weight Loss Intentions in Young Adults." *Obesity* 1157–62. Accessed August 2011. http://www.ncbi.nlm.nih.gov/pubmed/21164501.

2. "Weight Loss Possible When Self-Belief Is High." May 2, 2008. *ScienceDaily*, Accessed August 2011. http://www.sciencedaily.com/releases/2008/05/080502082735.htm.

3. Anderson, R., D. Anderson, and C. Hurst. October 2010. "Modeling Factors that Influence Exercise and Dietary Change among Midlife Australian Women: Results from the Healthy Aging of Women Study." *Maturitas* 67 (2): 151–58. Accessed August 2011. http://www.ncbi.nlm.nih.gov/pubmed/20619979.

4. Interview with Melissa Paris, Certified nutritionist and owner of Melissa Paris Fitness, New York City.

5. Schvey, Natasha A., R. M. Puhl, and K. D. Brownell. October 2011. "The Impact of Weight Stigma on Caloric Consumption." *Obesity* 19: 1957–1962. Accessed August 2011. http://www.nature.com/oby/journal/v19/n10/full/oby2011204a.html.

6. Interview with Christy D. Hofsess, PhD, Licensed psychologist and assistant professor in the Department of Counseling and Health Psychology, Bastyr University, Kenmore, WA.

7. Interview with Amy Wood, PsyD, A psychologist in private practice, in Portland, Maine, and author of *Life Your Way*.

8. Welsh, S., C. Davis, and A. Shaw. November/December 1992. "A Brief History of Food Guides in the United States." *Nutrition Today* 6–11.

Chapter 7

1. Hollis, Jack F. August 2008. "Weight-Loss during the Intensive Intervention Phase of the Weight-Loss Maintenance Trial." *American Journal of Preventive Medicine* 35 (2): 118–26. Accessed July 2011. http://www.ncbi.nlm.nih.gov/pmc/articles/PMC2515566/?tool=pubmed.

2. Center for Health Research. July 8, 2008. "CHR Study Finds Keeping Food Diaries Doubles Weight Loss." Kaiser Permanente. Accessed July 2011. http://www.kpchr.org/research/public/News.aspx?NewsID=3.

3. Interview with Theresa Piotrowski, MD, Medical director of the Medical and Surgical Weight Loss Center, The Lahey Clinic, Boston.

4. Interview with H. Theresa Wright, MS, RD, LDN, Founder of Renaissance Nutrition Center, Inc., East Norriton, PA.

5. Center for Health Research. August 18, 2010. "The More Frequently You Log On, the More Weight You Can Keep Off." Kaiser Permanente. Accessed July 2011. http://www.kpchr.org/research/public/News.aspx?NewsID=53.

6. Consumer Research. January 2010. "How to Buy a Bathroom Scale." Accessed July 2011. http://www.consumersearch.com/bathroom-scales/how-to-buy-a-bathroom-scale.

7. MayoClinic.com. "Is Sea Salt Better For Your Health Than Table Salt?" http://www.mayoclinic.com/health/sea-salt/AN01142.

Chapter 8

1. EverydayHealth.com. "Outrageous Diet Fads." http://www.everydayhealth.com/diet-and-nutrition-pictures/crazy-diet-fads.aspx.

2. Time.com. "A Brief History of Fad Diets." http://www.time.com/time/health/article/0,8599,1947605,00.html.

3. American Heart Association. "Quick Weight-Loss or Fad Diets." http://www.heart.org/HEARTORG/GettingHealthy/NutritionCenter/Quick-Weight-Loss-or-Fad-Diets_UCM_305970_Article.jsp.

4. American Diabetes Association (ADA). "Does Eating Breakfast Really Help with Weight Loss?" http://www.eatright.org/Public/content.aspx?id=6442453049&terms=breakfast.

5. ADA. "Make Time for Breakfast." http://www.eatright.org/kids/article.aspx?id=6442462528&terms=breakfast.

6. ADA. "Breakfast: The Right Start Every Day." http://www.eatright.org/Public/content.aspx?id=3759&terms=breakfast+and+blood+sugar.

7. Wyatt, H. R., G. K. Grunwald, C. L. Mosca, M. L. Klem, R. R. Wing, and J. O. Hill. February 2002. "Long-Term Weight Loss and Breakfast in Subjects in the National Weight-Control Registry." *Obesity Research*. Accessed July 2011. http://www.ncbi.nlm.nih.gov/pubmed/11836452.

8. Timlin, M. T., M. A. Pereira, M. Story, and D. Neumark-Sztainer. March 2008. "Breakfast Eating and Weight Change in a Five-Year Prospective Analysis of Adolescents: Project EAT." *Pediatrics*. Accessed July 2011. http://www.ncbi.nlm.nih.gov/pubmed/18310183.

9. ADA. "Want to Trim Your Waist? Try Eating Breakfast!" http://www.eatright.org/Media/Blog.aspx?id=4294969065&blogid=269&terms=breakfast.

10. Interview with Lisa Bunce, RD, Owner of Back to Basics Nutrition Consulting, in Redding, CT, who developed the My Lil'Coach app at www.mylilcoach.com.

11. Interview with Bonnie Taub-Dix, RD, Owner of BTD Nutrition Consultants, in New York City and Long Island and author of *Read It Before You Eat It*.

12. Clegg, M., and A. Shafat. 2010. "Gastric Emptying and Orocaecal Transit Time of Meals Containing Lactulose or Insulin in Men." *British Journal of Nutrition*. http://www.ncbi.nlm.nih.gov/pubmed/20370945.

13. ADA. "Eat Like a Bird, But…," http://www.eatright.org/nnm/blog.aspx?id= 6442451240&blogid=6442450952&terms=mini+meals.

14. Hamedani, Atyeh., T. Akhavan, G. H. Anderson, and R. A. Samra. May 2009. "Reduced Energy Intake at Breakfast is Not Compensated For at Lunch if a High-Insoluble-Fiber Cereal Replaces a Low-Fiber Cereal." *American Journal of Clinical Nutrition* 89 (5). Accessed July 2011. http://www.ajcn.org/content/89/5/1343.abstract.

15. Epiphaniou, Eleni, and Ogden, Jane. September 2010. "Successful Weight Loss Maintenance and a Shift in Identity from Restriction to a New Liberated Self." *Journal of Health Psychology.* Accessed July 2011. http://hpq.sagepub.com/content/15/6/887.abstractA.

16. Fletcher, Dan. December 15, 2009. "A Brief History of Fad Diets." *Time.*

17. http://www.cdc.gov/obesity/data/trends.html.

18. http://www.eatright.org/Public/content.aspx?id=6442460382&terms =food+combiningh.

19. http://www.webmd.com/diet/guide/low-calorie-diets.

Chapter 9

1. Interview with Lisa Bunce, RD, Owner of Back to Basics Nutrition Consulting, in Redding, CT, who developed the My Lil'Coach app at www.mylilcoach.com.

2. Paddon-Jones, D., E. Westman, R. D. Mattes, R. R. Wolfe, A. Astrup, and M. Westerterp-Plantenga. May 2008. "Protein, Weight Management, and Satiety." *American Journal of Clinical Nutrition.* Accessed May 2011. http://www.ajcn.org/content/87/5/1558S.full.

3. Interview with Jessica Levinson, MS, RD, Owner of Nutritioulicious, a nutrition counseling and consulting practice, New York City.

4. Fulgoni III, Victor L. May 2008. "Current Protein Intake in America: Analysis of the National Health and Nutrition Examination Survey, 2003–2004." *American Journal of Clinical Nutrition.* Accessed May 2011. http://www.ajcn.org/content/87/5/1554S.full.

5. ADA. "The Power of Protein." http://www.eatright.org/Public/content. aspx?id=6442460042&terms=protein.

6. ADA. "Whole-Grain Shopping List, Wheat Foods Council." http://www. wheatfoods.org/Resource-ShoppingList/Index.htm.

7. ADA. "Lean Meats." http://www.diabetes.org/food-and-fitness/food/ what-can-i-eat/meat-and-plant-based-protein.html.

8. ADA. "Fat and Diabetes." http://www.diabetes.org/food-and-fitness/food/what-can-i-eat/fat-and-diabetes.html.

9. Interviews with nutritionists and from the *Eat Right Nutrition Tips*, The American Dietetic Association: http://www.eatright.org/Public/content.aspx?id=206.

10. American Dietetic Association. "Color Your Plate with Salad." http://www.eatright.org/Public/content.aspx?id=206.

11. American Dietetic Association. "Whip Up a Homemade Salad Dressing." http://www.eatright.org/Public/content.aspx?id=6442452414&terms=salad+dressing.

Chapter 10

1. American Heart Association. "Saturated Fats." http://www.heart.org/HEARTORG/GettingHealthy/FatsAndOils/Fats101/Saturated-Fats_UCM_301110_Article.jsp.

2. Fung, Teresa T., R. M. van Dam, S. E. Hankinson, M. Stampfer, W. C. Willett, F. B. Hu. September 7, 2010. "Low-Carbohydrate Diets and All-Cause and Cause-Specific Mortality" *Annals of Internal Medicine* 153 (5). Accessed May 2011. http://www.annals.org/content/153/5/289.abstract.

3. Harvard School of Public Health. "Source: Protein—Expert Answers to Readers' Questions." http://www.hsph.harvard.edu/nutritionsource/questions/protein-questions/index.html#howmuch.

4. Nitrates and Nitrites, Ohio Bureau of Environmental Health, pdf.

5. American Heart Association. "Vegetarian Diets." http://www.american-heart.org/presenter.jhtml?identifier=4777.

6. CalorieKing: http://www.calorieking.com/foods/calories-in-beef-steak-organic-prairie-new-york-strip-boneless-frozen_f-ZmlkPTkxMjIz.html.

7. CalorieKing: http://www.calorieking.com/foods/calories-in-fresh-fish-cod-atlantic-pacific-cooked-dry-heat_f-ZmlkPTcwNjk0.html.

8. CalorieKing: http://www.calorieking.com/foods/calories-in-sausages-italian-pork-cooked_f-ZmlkPTcwMjA2.html.

9. Shahar D. R., D. Schwarzfuchs, D Fraser, et al. "Dairy Calcium Intake, Serum Vitamin D, and Successful Weight Loss." *American Journal of Clinical Nutrition*. Accessed September 1, 2010. http://www.ajcn.org/content/early/2010/09/01/ajcn.2010.29355.abstract.

10. "Soy and Health." Physicians Committee for Responsible Medicine, pdf.

11. American Institute for Cancer Research. "The New American Plate: Science-Based Approach." http://www.aicr.org/site/PageServer?pagename=reduce_diet_new_american_plate_science.

12. http://www.americangrassfedbeef.com/grass-fed-beef-jerky.asp.

13. National Institutes of Health. "Dietary Supplement Fact Sheet: Calcium, Office of Dietary Supplements." http://ods.od.nih.gov/factsheets/calcium.

14. CalorieKing: http://www.calorieking.com/foods/calories-in-sausages-turkey-cooked_f-ZmlkPTk1NjA2.html.

15. Food and Drug Administration. "Mercury Levels in Commercial Fish and Shellfish." http://www.fda.gov/Food/FoodSafety/Product-SpecificInformation/Seafood/FoodbornePathogensContaminants/Methylmercury/ucm115644.htm.

16. Crystal Petrello

17. "More Protein, Less Refined Starch Important for Dieting, Large Study Shows." *ScienceDaily*, http://www.sciencedaily.com/releases/2010/11/101124171536.htm.

18. "Soy and Health." Physicians Committee for Responsible Medicine, pdf.

19. Harvard School of Public Health. "The Nutrition Source: Protein—Moving Closer to Center Stage." http://www.hsph.harvard.edu/nutritionsource/what-should-you-eat/protein-full-story/index.html.

Chapter 11

1. Interview with Jessica Levinson, MS, RD, Owner of Nutritioulicious, a nutrition counseling and consulting practice, New York City.

2. Schoeller, D. A., and A. C. Buchholz. May 2005. "Energetics of Obesity and Weight Control: Does diet composition matter?" *Journal of the American Dietetic Association* 105. http://www.ncbi.nlm.nih.gov/pubmed/15867892.

3. Mayo Clinic. "Dietary Fats: Know Which Types to Choose." http://www.mayoclinic.com/health/fat/NU00262.

4. "Long-Term, High-Fat Diet Alters Mice Brains: Brain Changes May Contribute to Cycles of Weight Gain." January 19, 2011. *ScienceDaily*, Accessed May 2011. http://www.sciencedaily.com/releases/2010/11/101115112727.htm.

5. American Heart Association. "Know Your Fats." http://www.heart.org/HEARTORG/Conditions/Cholesterol/PreventionTreatmentofHighCholesterol/Know-Your-Fats_UCM_305628_Article.jsp.

6. CalorieKing, large egg, http://www.calorieking.com/foods/calories-in-eggs-chicken-egg-whole-hard-boiled_f-ZmlkPTExMjk.html.

7. CalorieKing, peanut butter, http://www.calorieking.com/foods/calories-in-nut-spreads-peanut-butter-smooth-style-with-salt_f-ZmlkPTgyNjU1.html.

8. National Heart Lung and Blood Institute. "Low-Calorie, Lower Fat Alternative Foods." National Institutes of Health, http://www.nhlbi.nih.gov/health/public/heart/obesity/lose_wt/lcal_fat.htm.

9. http://pubs.acs.org/cen/whatstuff/stuff/8233margarine.html.

Chapter 12

1. Interview with Judy Simon, RD, Clinical dietitian, The University of Washington Family Medicine.

2. Howarth, N. C., T. T. Huang, S. B. Roberts, and M. A. McCrory. September 2005. "Dietary Fiber and Fat are Associated with Excess Weight in Young and Middle-aged US Adults." *Journal of the American Dietetic Association* 105. Accessed June 2011. http://www.ncbi.nlm.nih.gov/pubmed/16129077.

3. Flood-Obbagy, Julie E., and Barbara J. Rolls. April 2009. "The Effect of Fruit in Different Forms on Energy Intake and Satiety at a Meal." *Appetite* 52 (2). Accessed June 2011. http://www.sciencedirect.com/science/article/pii/S019566630800620X.

4. CalorieKing.com.

5. MayoClinic. "Dietary Fiber: Essential for a Healthy Diet." http://www.mayoclinic.com/health/fiber/NU00033.

6. Harvard School of Public Health. "The Nutrition Source: Fiber: Start Roughing It!" http://www.hsph.harvard.edu/nutritionsource/what-should-you-eat/fiber-full-story/index.html.

7. Harvard School of Public Health. "The Nutrition Source: Fiber." http://www.hsph.harvard.edu/nutritionsource/what-should-you-eat/fiber/

8. U.S. Department of Agriculture MyPlate. "What Foods Are in the Grains Group?" http://www.choosemyplate.gov/foodgroups/grains.html.

9. Whole Grain Council. "Cooking Whole Grains." http://www.wholegrainscouncil.org/recipes/cooking-whole-grains.

10. Whole Grains Council. "Easy Ways to Enjoy Whole Grains." http://www.wholegrainscouncil.org/whole-grains-101/easy-ways-to-enjoy-whole-grains.

Chapter 13

1. Interview with Kate Hawley, RD, Clinical dietitian at Maine Medical Center, Portland, Maine.

2. Crystal Petrello

3. Horswill, Craig A., and Lynne M. Janas. August 2011. "Hydration and Health." *American Journal of Lifestyle Medicine* 5 (4): 304–15. Accessed July 2011. http://ajl.sagepub.com/content/5/4/304.abstract.

4. "Clinical Trial Confirms Effectiveness of Simple Appetite Control Method." August 23, 2010. *American Chemical Society* Press Release. Accessed July 2011, http://portal.acs.org/portal/acs/corg/content?_nfpb=true&_pageLabel=PP_ARTICLEMAIN&node_id=222&content_id=CNBP_025391&use_sec=true&sec_url_var=region1&__uuid=4fd02497-8c2a-4ab3-8269-9fadfc7f8065.

5. CalorieKing.com.

6. Boschmann, Michael., J. Steiniger, U. Hille, J. Tank, F. Adams, A. M. Sharma, S. Klaus, F. C. Luft, and J. Jordan. December 1, 2003. "Water-Induced Thermogenesis." *The Journal of Clinical Endocrinology & Metabolism* 88 (12). Accessed July 2011. http://jcem.endojournals.org/content/88/12/6015.abstract.

7. Institute of Medicine of the National Academy of Sciences. "Dietary Reference Intakes: Water, Potassium, Sodium, Chloride, and Sulfate." February 11, 2004. Accessed July 2011. http://www.iom.edu/Reports/2004/Dietary-Reference-Intakes-Water-Potassium-Sodium-Chloride-and-Sulfate.aspx.

8. Harvard School of Public Health. "The Nutrition Source: Ask the Expert: Coffee and Health." http://www.hsph.harvard.edu/nutritionsource/questions/coffee/

9. Starbucks Nutrition Information, http://www.starbucks.com/menu/catalog/nutrition?drink=all#view_control=nutrition&drink=bottled-drinks&drink=brewed-coffee&drink=chocolate&drink=espresso&drink=frappuccino-blended-beverages&drink=kids-drinks-and-other&drink=tazo-tea&drink=vivanno-smoothies.

10. Rolls, B. J. February 2010. "Plenary Lecture 1: Dietary Strategies for the Prevention and Treatment of Obesity." *Proceedings of the Nutrition Society* 69 (1). Accessed July 2011. http://www.ncbi.nlm.nih.gov/pubmed/19954563.

11. Flood J. E., and B. J. Rolls. November 2007. "Soup Preloads in a Variety of Forms Reduce Meal Energy Intake." *Appetite* 49 (3): 626–34. Accessed July 2011. http://www.ncbi.nlm.nih.gov/pubmed/17574705.

12. PubMed Health. "Hyponatremia." http://www.ncbi.nlm.nih.gov/pubmedhealth/PMH0001431/

13. Centers for Disease Control and Prevention. "Low-Energy-Dense Foods and Weight Management: Cutting Calories While Controlling

Hunger." http://www.cdc.gov/nccdphp/dnpa/nutrition/pdf/r2p_energy_d.

14. http://stopsportsinjuries.reingoldweb.com/files/pdf/ACSM-position-statement-Exertional-Heat-Illness.pdf

15. Dunford, Marie (Ed.). Sports Nutrition: A Practice Manual for Professionals, 4th edition. Amer Dietetic Assn, September 2006.

Chapter 14

1. Calgon commercial: http://www.youtube.com/watch?v=WVf1lClfBng.

2. "Everyday Stress Linked to Obesity." September 2, 2010. University of Cincinnati press release, Accessed July 2011. http://healthnews.uc.edu/news/?/11289/

3. "Stress May Cause Excess Abdominal Fat in Otherwise Slender Women, Study Conducted At Yale Shows." November 23, 2000. *ScienceDaily*. Accessed July 2011. http://www.sciencedaily.com/releases/2000/11/001120072314.htm.

4. MayoClinic.com. "Stress: Constant Stress Puts Your Health at Risk." http://www.mayoclinic.com/health/stress/SR00001.

5. Interview with Amy Wood, PsyD, A psychologist in private practice, in Portland, Maine, and author of *Life Your Way*.

6. American Psychological Association. "Mind/Body Health: Obesity." http://www.apa.org/helpcenter/obesity.aspx.

7. The American Institute of Stress. "America's No. 1 Health Problem: Why Is There More Stress Today?" http://www.stress.org/americas.htm?AIS=81e46698ca819b9467ed323d551685fe.

8. Epel, Elissa S., B. McEwen, T. Seeman, K. Matthews, G. Castellazzo, K. D. Brownell, J. Bell, and J. R. Ickovics. September 1, 2000. "Stress and Body Shape: Stress-Induced Cortisol Secretion Is Consistently Greater Among Women with Central Fat." *Psychosomatic Medicine* 62 (5): 623–32. Accessed July 2011. http://www.psychosomaticmedicine.org/content/62/5/623.full.

9. American Psychological Association. 2010. "Stress in America: Key Findings." http://www.apa.org/news/press/releases/stress/key-findings.aspx.

10. American Heart Association. "Four Ways to Deal with Stress." http://www.heart.org/HEARTORG/GettingHealthy/StressManagement/

FourWaystoDealWithStress/Four-Ways-to-Deal-with-Stress_UCM_
307996_Article.jsp.

11. Hahn, I. H., M. B. Grynderup, S. B. Dalsgaard, J. F.Thomsen, A. M. Hansen,
     A. Kaergaard, L. Kaerlev, et al. March 1, 2011. "Does Outdoor Work During
     the Winter Season Protect Against Depression and Mood Difficulties?"
     Scandinavian Journal of Work, Environment&Health. Accessed July 2011. http://
     www.ncbi.nlm.nih.gov/pubmed/21359494.

12. MayoClinic.com. "Depression and Anxiety: Exercise Eases Symptoms."
     http://www.mayoclinic.com/health/depression-and-exercise/
     MH00043.

13. MayoClinic.com. "Tai Chi: The Many Possible Health Benefits." http://
     www.mayoclinic.com/health/tai-chi/SA00087/METHOD=print.

14. Lai, H. L., C. J. Chen,T. C. Peng, F. M. Chang, M. L. Hsieh, H.Y. Huang, and
     S. C. Chang. February 2006. "Randomized ControlledTrial of Music During
     Kangaroo Care on Maternal State Anxiety and Preterm Infants' Responses."
     International Journal of Nursing Studies 43 (2): 139–46. Accessed July 2011.
     http://www.ncbi.nlm.nih.gov/pubmed?term=Randomized%20
     controlled%20trial%20of%20music%20during%20kangaroo%20
     care%20on%20maternal%20state%20anxiety%20and%20preterm%
     20infants'%20responses.

15. National Center for Complementary and Alternative Medicine. "Long-
     Term Yoga Practice May Decrease Women's Stress." http://nccam.nih.
     gov/research/results/spotlight/051510.htm.

16. MayoClinic.com. "Relaxation Techniques: Try These Steps to Reduce
     Stress." http://www.mayoclinic.com/health/relaxation-technique/
     SR00007/METHOD=print.

17. American Psychological Association. "StressTip Sheet." http://www.apa.
     org/news/press/releases/2007/10/stress-tips.aspx.

18. Martens, M. J., F. Rutters, S. G. Lemmens, J. M. Born, and M. S. Westerterp-
     Plantenga. December 2, 2010. "Effects of Single Macronutrients on Serum
     Cortisol Concentrations in Normal Weight Men," *Physiology & Behavior*
     101 (5): 563–67. Accessed July 2011. http://www.ncbi.nlm.nih.gov/
     pubmed/20849868.

19. American Psychological Association. "Mind/Body Health: Stress." http://
     www.apa.org/helpcenter/stress.aspx.

20. American Psychological Association. "Overwhelmed by Workplace
     Stress?You're Not Alone." http://www.apa.org/helpcenter/work-stress.
     aspx.

21. "Sleep to Live." *Sleep Training Manual,* April 29, 2010.

Chapter 15

1. Interview with Robert Oexman, DC, Director of the Sleep to Live Institute, Joplin, MO.
2. "Sleep to Live." *Sleep Training Manual*, April 29, 2010.
3. Chaput, Jean-Philippe., J. P. Després, C. Bouchard, and A. Tremblay. April 1, 2008. "The Association between Sleep Duration and Weight Gain in Adults: A 6-Year Prospective Study from the Quebec Family Study." *Sleep* 31 (4). Accesed June 2011. http://www.journalsleep.org/ViewAbstract.aspx?pid=27117.
4. Nedeltcheva, Arlet V., J. M. Kilkus, J. Imperial, K. Kasza, D. A. Schoeller, and P. D. Penev. January 2009. "Sleep Curtailment Is Accompanied by Increased Intake of Calories from Snacks." *American Journal of Clinical Nutrition* 89 (1). Accessed June 2011. http://www.ncbi.nlm.nih.gov/pmc/articles/PMC2615460/?tool=pubmed.
5. "Annual Sleep in America Poll Exploring Connections with Communications Technology Use and Sleep." National Sleep Foundation press release. March 7, 2011. Accessed June 2011. http://www.sleepfoundation.org/article/press-release/annual-sleep-america-poll-exploring-connections-communications-technology-use-
6. National Sleep Foundation. "Poll Reveals Sleep Differences among Ethnic Groups." http://www.sleepfoundation.org/article/press-release/poll-reveals-sleep-differences-among-ethnic-groups.
7. National Sleep Foundation. "Obesity and Sleep." http://www.sleepfoundation.org/article/sleep-topics/obesity-and-sleep.
8. Interview with Sheila Abrahams, a yoga instructor based in Hernando, FL, and adjunct professor of nutrition, College of Central Florida.
9. MayoClinic. "Acupuncture: Definition." http://www.mayoclinic.com/health/acupuncture/MY00946.
10. Ernst, E., M. S. Lee, and T. Y. Choi. June 2011. "Acupuncture for Insomnia? An Overview of Systematic Reviews." *European Journal of General Practice* 17 (2): 116–23. Accessed June 2011. http://www.ncbi.nlm.nih.gov/pubmed/21463162.
11. Stanford School of Medicine. February 8, 2011. "Study of Acupuncture as Sleep Therapy for Breast-cancer Survivors Seeks Participants." http://med.stanford.edu/ism/2011/february/acupuncture.html.
12. Freire, A. O., G. C. Sugai, S. M. Togeiro, L. E. Mello, and S. Tufik. September 2010. "Immediate Effect of Acupuncture on the Sleep Pattern of Patients with Obstructive Sleep Apnea." *Acupuncture in Medicine*

28 (3): 115–19. Accessed June 2011. http://www.ncbi.nlm.nih.gov/pubmed/20615853.

13. American Cancer Society. "Biofeedback." http://www.cancer.org/Treatment/TreatmentsandSideEffects/ComplementaryandAlternative-Medicine/MindBodyandSpirit/biofeedback.

14. Cleveland Clinic. "Biofeedback for Sleep Disorders." http://my.clevelandclinic.org/Documents/Sleep_Disorders_Center/Biofeedback.pdf.

15. http://www.askdrsears.com/topics/family-nutrition/foods-sleep/foods-help-you-sleep.

16. http://www.umm.edu/altmed/articles/melatonin-000315.htm.

17. http://www.sleepfoundation.org/article/sleep-topics/food-and-sleep.

18. http://www.webmd.com/vitamins-and-supplements/lifestyle-guide-11/natural-good-sleep-tips-on-melatonin-valerian?page=1.

Chapter 16

1. Interview with Keri Gans, RD, Author of The Small-Change Diet and a nutritionist in private practice, New York City.

2. Interview with Jo Ann Hattner, RD, Author of Gut Insight and a dietitian in private practice, San Francisco.

3. Interview with Robert A. Gabbay, MD, PhD, An endocrinologist and director of the Diabetes and Obesity Institute, Pennsylvania State Hershey Medical Center.

4. Based on several What Works for Me interviews.

5. Interview with Amy Wood, PsyD, A psychologist in private practice in Portland, Maine, and author of Life Your Way.

6. National Weight Control Registry. "NWCR Facts." http://www.nwcr.ws/Research/default.htm.

7. Broom, David R., R. L. Batterham, J. A. King, and D. J. Stensel. January 2009. "Influence of Resistance and Aerobic Exercise on Hunger, Circulating Levels of Acylated Ghrelin, and Peptide YY in Healthy Males." American Journal of Physiology 296 (1). Accessed August 2011. http://ajpregu.physiology.org/content/296/1/R29.full.

8. Interview with Kate Hawley, RD, Clinical dietitian at Maine Medical Center, Portland, Maine.

9. "Out of Body Image." Ms. Magazine, Spring 2008. http://www.msmagazine.com/spring2008/outOfBodyImage.asp.

Index